Behçet's Disease

Yoshiaki Ishigatsubo
Editor

Behçet's Disease

From Genetics to Therapies

Springer

Editor
Yoshiaki Ishigatsubo
Department of Internal Medicine and Clinical Immunology
Yokohama City University Graduate School of Medicine
Yokohama, Japan

ISBN 978-4-431-54486-9 ISBN 978-4-431-54487-6 (eBook)
DOI 10.1007/978-4-431-54487-6
Springer Tokyo Heidelberg New York Dordrecht London

Library of Congress Control Number: 2014956563

Printed on acid-free paper

Springer is part of Springer Science+Business Media (www.springer.com)

Preface

The pathogenesis of Behçet's disease, a rare and poorly understood condition causing mainly inflammation of the blood vessels, has been unknown for a long time, with most experts regarding it as an autoimmune and/or autoinflammatory condition. However, as the fields of technology, genetic epidemiology, and internal medicine evolve, recent achievements in the Genome-Wide Association Study (GWAS) have brought us abundant new insights into the pathogenesis of Behçet's disease. More specifically, whole genome association study results elucidating polymorphisms that implicate a relationship between many genes in the disease pathogenicity, other than human leukocyte antigen, have been reported by groups from Yokohama City University, the National Institutes of Health, and Istanbul University. Cooperative efforts between these institutions are ongoing, with attempts to analyze the functions of loci relevant to Behçet's disease and associated symptoms currently under way. This cooperative endeavor adds special value to this book.

Regarding progress in the clinical field, a practical guideline for the treatment of systemic disorders such as vascular, neural, or intestinal lesions in Behçet's disease has been requested for long time. Despite much ongoing research in this field and advances in medications for treatment options, we are still left with providing treatment for the symptoms and not the etiology of Behçet's disease. Because it is sometimes difficult to make a diagnosis, the prognoses of patients with those disorders are not usually good. In terms of treatment, an immunosuppressant or prednisone mainly has been administered for intractable uveitis and systemic types of the disorder with vascular, neural, or intestinal lesions in Behçet's disease. However, the outcome of the treatment with these medicines has been insufficient. Recently, therapy utilizing molecular targeted treatment has proven to be effective for many intractable diseases such as rheumatoid arthritis, systemic lupus erythematosus, inflammatory intestinal diseases, and so on throughout the world.

In a similar way, cytokine-targeting therapies, such as tumor necrosis factor (TNF) has been recently introduced for patients with Behçet's disease. For example, infliximab and adalimumab, monoclonal antibodies against tumor necrosis factor alpha (TNF-α), were approved for use in severe uveitis and intestinal Behçet's disease after clinical trials sponsored by the Japanese Ministry of Health, Labour and Welfare in 2007 and 2013, respectively. A post-marketing survey revealed that infliximab therapy in intractable uveitis decreased the frequency of the attack and, more surprisingly, ameliorated even visual acuity. There are also many reports showing the therapeutic efficacy of molecular targeted therapy with such biological agents as TNF-α, IL-6, and IL-1 inhibitors in intractable cases, including systemic disorders with vascular, neural, or intestinal lesions in Behçet's disease. Indeed, various clinical trials of therapy with molecular targeted treatment in Behçet's disease are now under way.

Advances in genetics are influencing our understanding of disease as discoveries about the human genome and their relevance to manifestations of disease and clinical symptoms are rapidly becoming an integral part of medical practice as well as having implications for translating basic research into translational medicine. Therefore, this book is not intended to cover every aspect of Behçet's disease. Instead, the book is organized to incorporate the latest advances and reflect the concepts that are relevant to clinical–pathologic correlation and the diagnosis of Behçet's disease. This book focuses on new topics in immunology and genetic findings, which have attracted the attention of many investigators for a variety of reasons. To that end, I invited the most active specialists among members of the Japanese Behçet's disease study group in various fields to write each chapter, in which they distilled and dispensed their clinical wisdom.

As previously mentioned, this book covers new ground by including up-to-date immunological and genetic advances in the diagnosis and treatment of Behçet's disease, further defining, and supporting the role of immunology and that of genomic analysis in clinical medicine. Evolving advances in information technology will aid readers by providing greater options for gaining access to this valuable information, reliably promoting international dissemination and acceptance. Because Behçet's disease afflicts individuals in more than one location around the world, it is my hope that practitioners, health professionals, medical educators, and medical students everywhere will benefit from the information contained herein for the good of patients, and that this latest information will be readily available as an indispensable clinical and medical education reference tool.

Among clinical findings, we have focused attention on the eyes (uveitis), because of the effect on the quality of life, and systemic disorders such as vascular, neural, or intestinal lesions, which affect the life prognosis. Therefore, this book also includes the new medical treatment guidelines proposed by the Japanese Behçet's disease study group based on the latest data. However, because Behçet's disease is an orphan disease, there are few specific case reports based on evidence-based medicine. Guidelines have been worked out based on the summary of opinions from the members of the Japanese Behçet's disease study group referring to case reports and questionnaires. It will be necessary to consider extensive feedback and comprehensive review of input and information in the future.

I would like to introduce this book so that it will be widely used by clinicians, medical students, and basic researchers who are interested in Behçet's disease. What started out years ago as a desire to communicate, collaborate, publish, and share information for improvement in understanding, treatment, and further study of Behçet's disease has led to this book. As no text is without shortcomings, I offer appreciation to our colleagues for feedback, comments, and ideas that might contribute to ongoing and future efforts toward understanding and treating Behçet's disease, and I welcome your suggestions.

Finally, I wish to express my appreciation to my associates, colleagues, and contributors who shared their knowledge, making this publication possible. I am especially grateful to the authors of each chapter, who have tirelessly and willingly devoted their time, energy, and expertise to this important endeavor. I am also appreciative of the contributions and support from members of the Behçet's disease study group, the Ministry of Health, Labour and Welfare in Japan, and I also extend my gratitude to the Japanese Behçet's Disease Patients' Society for providing many specimens for the study of Behçet's disease.

Yokohama, Japan Yoshiaki Ishigatsubo

Contents

Chapter 1
Overview

Yoshiaki Ishigatsubo and Mitsuhiro Takeno

Abstract Behçet's disease is an inflammatory disorder characterized by recurrent oral aphthae, genital ulcers, uveitis, and skin lesions such as erythema nodosum. Although mucocutaneous manifestations are self-limiting, ocular involvement can cause blindness. Involvement of large vessels, gastrointestinal tract, and central nervous system is less frequent but can be life-threatening and leave irreversible damage.

Because of heterogeneity of clinical manifestations, a number of sets of diagnostic or classification criteria have been proposed and are still being discussed. The most common causes of Behçet's disease related death are the arterial lesions, especially pulmonary arterial aneurysm, followed by chronic progressive neurological involvement. Introduction of anti-TNF mAb has greatly contributed to improvement of visual prognosis. Treatment with biologics, including TNF blockers, is also promising for other serious clinical subtypes.

Although the etiology remains unknown, both genetic and environmental factors are implicated in the development of the disease. In addition to the unique geographic distribution and familial aggregation of BD patients, recent gene-wide association studies and subsequent detail analyses have identified novel susceptible genes which are related to the immune system besides *HLA-B51*.

Keywords Silk Road disease • Prevalence • Familial clustering • Diagnostic criteria • Classification criteria • ISG criteria • ICBD criteria • Infliximab • Adalimumab

1.1 Introduction

Hulusi Behçet, a Turkish dermatologist, reported three patients with a triple symptom complex of aphthae, genital ulcers, and hypopyon uveitis in 1937 [1]. The name of Behçet's disease (BD) originated from this report. However, the disease is also called "Adamantides-Behçet's disease" in German, because Benediktos Adamantides had reported a patient who presented with various clinical

Y. Ishigatsubo, M.D., Ph.D. (✉) • M. Takeno
Department of Internal Medicine and Clinical Immunology, Yokohama City University Graduate School of Medicine, 3-9 Fukuura, Kanazawa-Ku, Yokohama 236-0004, Japan
e-mail: ishigats@med.yokohama-cu.ac.jp

Y. Ishigatsubo (ed.), *Behçet's Disease*,
DOI 10.1007/978-4-431-54487-6_1

manifestations like BD in 1930. Moreover, Hippocrates of Cos had already described the association of oral ulcers, genital ulcers, ocular lesions, and skin lesions, all of which were compatible with clinical manifestations of BD.

BD is now recognized as an inflammatory disorder characterized by recurrent oral aphthae, genital ulcers, uveitis, and skin lesions such as erythema nodosum [2]. All these common symptoms are recurrently episodic and self-limiting except ocular involvement can cause blindness. Indeed, BD had been the second most common cause of blindness in adults over the last century. Details of skin and ocular lesions are described in Chaps. 8 and 4, respectively. In addition, the disease has a broad spectrum of clinical phenotypes including involvement of large vessels, central nervous system (CNS), and gastrointestinal tract. These organ lesions are less frequent, but can be life-threatening and leave irreversible damage. Details are described in Chaps. 5, 6, and 7. Standard therapeutic strategies for various manifestations have not been established yet, though several sets of recommendations for management of BD had been released by EULAR in 2008 [3, 4] and others [5–7].

The etiology remains unknown, though both genetic and environmental factors are implicated in development of BD. The underlying pathology is vascular damages. In the 2012 Revised International Chapel Hill Consensus Conference Nomenclature of Vasculitides, BD is classified as variable vessel vasculitis [8], because the disease can affect vessels of any size and type.

During the last decade, we have had two major progressions in this field. First, advanced molecular technology leads to new insights of genetic predisposition. In 2010, gene-wide association studies (GWAS) identified *IL10* and *IL12RB-IL23R* as susceptible genes besides *HLAB51* in two independent patient populations, Japan and Turkey [9, 10]. The replication studies covered in BD patients from almost all prevalent areas. The GWAS has been the breakthrough in the pathogenesis of BD. Subsequently, a series of genetic analyses have identified novel susceptible genes [11–15], most of which are involved in innate and acquired immune abnormalities. Details are described in Chaps. 2 and 3.

Another progression is the introduction of antitumor necrosis factor (TNF)-α mAb for uveitis in BD patients [7, 16–19]. The therapy has contributed to the improvement of visual outcome in the patients. Moreover, several reports have shown that anti-TNF therapies are effective for intestinal [20–22], CNS [23], and large vascular lesions [24, 25] which are resistant to conventional treatment.

This overview mainly focuses on clinical issues including epidemiology, classification criteria, clinical course, and prognosis in BD.

1.2 Epidemiology

BD is often called "Silk Road disease," because the patients cluster along the ancient Silk Road, which extended from the Mediterranean area and Middle East Asia to Far East Asia [2]. A number of epidemiological studies have demonstrated regional differences in prevalence of BD (Table 1.1). Turkey has highest prevalence ranging from 20 to 421 per 100,000 adults (>10 or 12 y.o.), though onset in childhood is

Table 1.1 Prevalence of Behçet's disease in previous epidemiological studies

Author	Year	Country	Study area	Incidence (per 100,000)	Ethnic	Age
Asia						
Demirhindi [26]	1981	Turkey	Istanbul, rural	80.0		
Yurdakul [27]	1988	Turkey	Ordu, rural	370.0		
Idil [28]	2002	Turkey	Ankara, suburban	115.0		>10
Azizlerli [29]	2003	Turkey	Istanbul, urban	421.0		>12
Cakir [30]	2004	Turkey	Edirne, rural	20.0		
Jaber [48]	2002	Israel	Taibe, urban	120.0	Arabs	
Krause [49]	2007	Israel	Galilee	15.2	All	>15
				46.0	Jewish	
				49.0	Arabs	
				146.4	Druze	
Davatchi [33]	1997	Iran	Nationwide	16.7		
Davatchi [34]	2008	Iran	Tehran, urban	80.0		
Al-Rawi [35]	2003	Iraq	Saglawia	17.0		
Al-Dalaan [33]	1997	Saudi Arabia	Al Quassim	19.5		
Yamamoto [31]	1974	Japan	Nationwide	7.0–8.5		
Nakae [32]	1993	Japan	Nationwide	13.5		
	2012	Japan	Nationwide	14.6		
Mok [44]	2002	China	Hong Kong	2.6		
Chen [45]	2001	Taiwan		1.0		
Europe						
Crespo [33]	1993	Portugal	Coimbra, urban	1.5		
Sanchez Burson [33]	1998	Spain		7.5		
Gonzalez-Gay [36]	2000	Spain	Lugo (1988–1997)	6.4		
Grana [37]	2001	Spain	Galicia (1978–1990)	5.6		
Mahr [33]	2008	France	Seine-Saint-Denis	7.2		>15
		France	Seine-Saint-Denis	2.4	European	>15
Salvarani [38]	2007	Italy	Reggio-Emilia, rural	3.8		
Zouboulis [39]	1997	Germany	Berlin-West, urban	0.6	German	
Papoutis [40]	2006	Germany	Berlin-West, urban	1.47	German	
				26.6	Non-German	
				77.37	Turks	
Chamberlain [41]	1977	England	Yorkshire, rural	0.6		
Jankowski [42]	1992	Scotland	Nationwide	0.3		
Ek [43]	1993	Sweden	Nationwide	3.5	All	
				1.2	Swedish	
Others						
Hirohata [50]	1975	USA	Hawaii	0.0		
O'Duffy [46]	1978	USA	Olmsted, rural	0.3		
Assaad-Khalil [33]	1997	Egypt	Alexandria	7.6		

rare [26–30]. In Japan, the prevalence was 14.6 per 100,000 in 2012 according to the data of a national insurance system in which 18,636 patients with BD were registered, while it was 7.0–8.5 in 1974 [31] and 13.5 in 1993 [2, 32]. The prevalence per 100,000 individuals was reported as 16.7–80.0 in Iran [33, 34], 17 in Iraq [35], 19.5 in Saudi Arabia [33], and 7.6 in Egypt [33], whereas it was 0.27–7.5 in the European countries [33, 36–43], 2.6 in Hong Kong [44], 1.0 in Taiwan [45], and 0.33 in the United States [46].

A number of studies have shown significant association of BD with HLA-B51 in different ethnic groups. The association is stronger in the endemic areas than the other regions. The unique geographic distribution of the patients corresponds to the highest distribution of HLA-B51-positive individuals [47], though the finding does not exclude effects of environmental factors on the disease onset. It is helpful to study the prevalence of immigrants from endemic areas to non-endemic areas, when considering this issue. A population-based study in France showed that the prevalence of BD for European, North African, and Asian ancestry was 2.4, 34.6, and 17.5, respectively [33]. Similarly, in Berlin, the prevalence in Turkish immigrants was higher than that in Germany natives [33, 39]. Two independent studies from Israel showed that the prevalence was 15.2 among the ethnic Jews and 120 in an Arab community, indicating that ethnic origin is an important factor to determine the prevalence of BD [26, 48, 49]. These findings suggested that BD has a primarily hereditary basis. On the other hands, BD is rare among Japanese immigrants in Hawaii and California [50], suggesting that environmental factors also play a certain role in the disease.

The majority of BD patients are sporadic cases, though a positive family history was noted among 2–3 % of Japanese patients and 8–34 % of the Turkish and Middle East patients with BD [51]. In a familial study of 170 consecutive unrelated BD patients, sibling recurrence rate was calculated to be 4.2 % for BD and 13.3 % for recurrent oral ulcers, and the sibling recurrence ratio (λs) was ranged from 11.4 to 52.5 in Turkey [51]. Juvenile onset and HLA-B51 are more common in familial patients [52, 53]. Although shared environmental factors may have some contribution to familial clustering in part, these data support implication of genetic factors in BD. These underlying observations eventually led to recent studies such as GWAS and subsequent studies, which determined a number of novel susceptible genes (see Chap. 3).

BD appears most frequently in the third to fourth decade. Childhood and elderly onsets are rare. Ratio of gender is different among countries. While BD is more common among females in Japan and Korea, male patients are predominant in Middle Eastern countries [2]. Severe manifestations such as uveitis [54, 55] and involvement of CNS [56–58] and large vessels [59, 60] are found mainly in male patients.

1.3 Clinical Manifestations and Classification Criteria

Clinical manifestations are diverse and heterogeneous among BD patients (Table 1.2) [2, 29, 32, 39, 49, 56, 61, 62]. Major symptoms such as oral aphthosis, genital ulcers, skin lesions, and ocular lesions are common in patients from any

Table 1.2 Frequency of symptoms in epidemiological studies with more than 100 patients from various countries

Author	Year	Country	Patient number	OA	GU	Eye	Skin	Pathergy	Joint	Epididymitis	GI	CNS	Vessel
				Percentage of patients									
Sakane [2]	1972	Japan	2,031	96	72	67	83	75	54	6	25	13	7
Nakae [32]	1991	Japan	3,316	98	73	69	87	44	57	6	16	11	9
Ideguchi [56]	2010	Japan	412	100	73	65	88		48	6	10	13	8
Zouboulis [39]	1996	Germany	130	98	79	48	73	53	59	32	NA	NA	NA
Dilsen [2]	1993	Turkey	496	100	77	47	78	NA	47	NA	5	8	38
Azizlerli [29]	2003	Turkey	101	100	70	28	(40[a], 37[b])	69	32	NA	NA	NA	NA
Krause [49]	2007	Israel	112	100	68	53	41	44	70	NA	NA	12	18
Assaad-Khalil [61]	1997	Egypt	274	92	76	76	39	58	50	NA	NA	NA	NA
Kim [62]	1988	Korea	410	99	82	40	73	NA	31	NA	10	12	2

OA oral aphtha, *GU* genital ulcer, *NA* not available
[a]Folliculitis
[b]Erythema nodosum

Table 1.3 Criteria for the diagnosis of Behçet's disease. Criteria for the diagnosis of Behçet's disease by International Study Group [63]

Findings	Definition
Recurrent oral ulcerations	Minor aphthous, major aphthous, or herpetiform ulceration observed by physician or patient, which recurred at least 3 times in one 12-month period
Plus 2 of the following	
Recurrent genital ulceration	Aphthous ulceration or scarring observed by physician or patient
Eye lesion	Anterior uveitis, posterior uveitis, or cells in vitreous on slit lamp examination or retinal vasculitis observed by ophthalmologist
Skin lesions	Erythema nodosum observed by physician or patient, pseudofolliculitis or papulopustular lesions, or acneiform nodules observed by physician in postadolescent patients not on corticosteroids
Positive pathergy test	Test interpreted as positive by the physician at 24–48 h

Note: Findings are applicable if no other clinical explanation is present

country, though there are some regional differences in other symptoms. For example, gastrointestinal involvement is more common in Far Eastern Asia such as Japan, and Korea than in other countries, whereas lower frequency of large vascular lesions is noted in the regions.

There are neither pathognomonic symptoms nor laboratory findings in BD. Imaging findings and even histological findings are also nonspecific. Therefore, the diagnosis relies on the combination of symptoms. Many sets of diagnostic or classification criteria had been proposed and used in daily practice and research until the International Study Group (ISG) set the classification criteria in 1990 (Table 1.3) [63]. Recurrent oral ulceration is essential in the ISG criteria. In addition, any of two or more symptoms among recurrent genital ulcerations, eye lesions, skin lesions, and positive pathergy test are required to classify a patient as BD. The criteria have contributed to international comparison of particular findings among different studies.

However, several issues have been raised in clinical application of the criteria for daily practice. First, sensitivity of the ISG criteria is lower than many other sets of criteria, because organ involvement is not included [64]. Second, patients presenting with BD symptoms except oral aphtha are never diagnosed as BD according to the ISG. Though the number of such patients is small, it is not negligible [65]. Third, several reports have shown that frequency of positive pathergy test has been decreasing since the mid-1980s [66]. Therefore, the test is not always conducted in daily practice, in spite of the high diagnostic specificity [67, 68].

To overcome these problems, the International Team for the Revision of the International Criteria for Behçet's Disease has recently proposed a new set of criteria (ICBD criteria) based on clinical data from 2556 BD patients and 1,163 controls from 27 countries (Table 1.4) [69, 70]. The criteria include neurological and vascular manifestations in addition to mucocutaneous and ocular symptoms. Pathergy test is not included in the primary scoring system, but it is optional. The positive result is considered as one point. These features were similar to those in the Japan revised

Table 1.4 Criteria for the diagnosis of Behçet's disease. International criteria for Behçet's disease – point score system: scoring ≥4 indicates Behçet's disease

Sign/symptom	Points
Ocular lesions	2
Genital aphthosis	2
Oral aphthosis	2
Skin lesions	1
Neurological manifestations	1
Vascular manifestations	1
Positive pathergy test	1*

Pathergy test is optional, and the primary scoring system does not include pathergy testing. However, where pathergy testing is conducted, one extra point may be assigned for a positive result

criteria (1987) (Table 1.5, 2014, draft of minor revision) [55], because neurological and vascular manifestations are included in minor symptoms, and the pathergy test is listed as a supportive finding as well as HLA-B51. In a cohort study based on the revised criteria from Japan, the pathergy test was conducted in 120 of 412 patients (29 %), especially in those who had difficulty in making the diagnosis [55].

Because the new set of ICBD criteria has higher sensitivity than the ISG criteria, clinical application of the new criteria may lead to earlier diagnosis and treatment with beneficial outcomes. On the other hand, specificity is lower in the new ICBD criteria than the ISG criteria. Of note, the ISG criteria are set to classify established BD patients for a research purpose rather than clinical application. Thus, it is important to understand that the purpose is different between both sets of criteria.

1.4 Clinical Course – Evolution of the Disease

It is very important to understand clinical course of BD patients, because all clinical manifestations during the clinical course should be considered when any sets of diagnostic or classification criteria are applied. All symptoms do not appear simultaneously at the onset of BD. In general, individual symptoms are gradually accumulated during the clinical courses, resulting in full-blown clinical features which satisfy the diagnostic criteria [55] (Fig. 1.1).

Oral aphtha is the most common initial symptoms (Table 1.6). According to a cohort study which investigated 412 patients from 1991 to 2007 in Japan, oral aphtha had been found a mean of 7.2 ± 10.2 years before the diagnosis was made [55] (Table 1.6, Fig. 1.1). Fourteen percent of the patients had suffered from the symptoms for more than 20 years until diagnosis. On the other hand, genital ulcers, skin lesions, and eye symptoms appeared in up to one fourth of patients as initial symptoms, though they were found in 60–90 % all along the clinical course in Japanese patients [2, 32, 55] (Table 1.2). Rather, the diagnosis is made by appearance of these

Table 1.5 Criteria for the diagnosis of Behçet's disease. Japan revised criteria (2014, draft of minor revision)

1. Major findings
(1) Major symptoms
1) Recurrent oral aphthoid ulcer
2) Skin lesions
(a) Erythema nodosum-like eruption
(b) Superficial thrombophlebitis
(c) Pseudofolliculitis or papulopustular lesion
Reference finding: Skin hyperirritability
3) Ocular symptoms
(a) Iridocyclitis
(b) Chorioretinitis
(c) Residual lesions suggesting previous (a) and (b) as follows:
Posterior synechia, pigmentation on lens, chorioretinal atrophy, optic nerve atrophy, complicated cataract, secondary glaucoma, ocular phthisis
4) Genital ulcer
(2) Minor symptoms
1) Arthritis without deformity and ankylosis
2) Epididymitis
3) Gastrointestinal lesions such as ileocecal ulcers
4) Vascular lesions
5) Central nervous system lesion
(3) Disease subtypes
1) Complete type: having all four major symptoms during the course
2) Incomplete type: having
(a) Three major symptoms, or two major plus two minor symptoms
(b) Typical ocular symptoms plus the other one major symptom or two minor symptoms
3) Probable: having a part of major symptoms but not meeting incomplete type and repeating or exacerbating typical minor symptoms
4) Special type
(a) Intestinal type: confirm the lesions by endoscopic examinations
(b) Vascular type: classify into aneurysm, arterial obstruction, deep vein thrombosis, and pulmonary lesions
(c) Neurological type: classify into acute type having meningitis or brainstem encephalitis and chronic progressive type having psychiatric symptoms and neurological manifestations such as truncal ataxia
2. Laboratory tests
Supportive laboratory finding (not essential)
(1) Pathergy test
(2) Inflammatory reaction: elevated ESR, positive CRP, leukocytosis, hypercomplementemia
(3) Positive HLA-B51, A26
(4) Pathology of skin lesions: cellular infiltration, vasculitis
(5) Cerebrospinal fluid: pleocytosis and elevated IL-6, and MRI: flare high intensity and brainstem atrophy

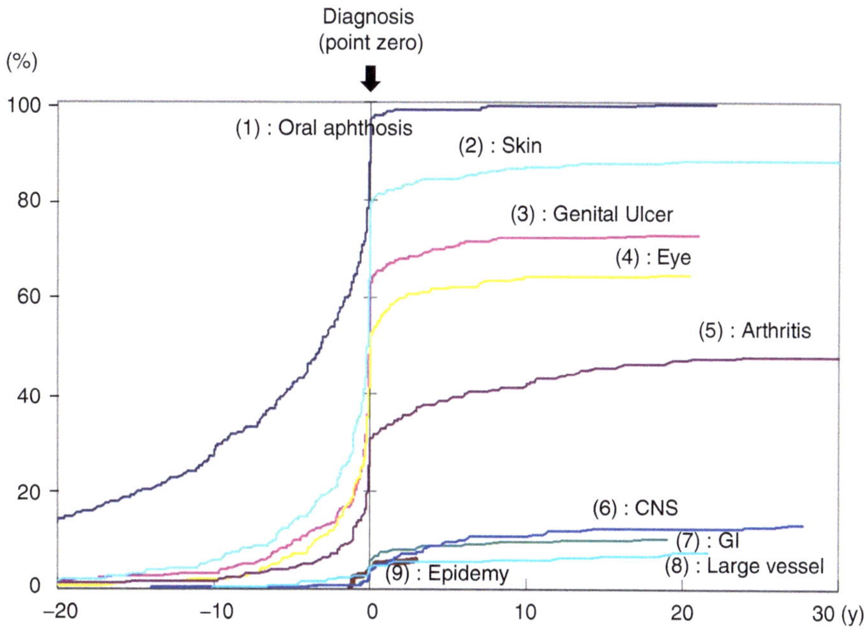

Fig. 1.1 Cumulative rate of appearance of each symptom ([55] with modification)
The zero point indicates the time of diagnosis based on the Japan revised criteria (1987). Negative value of the vertical axis indicates that symptoms precede the diagnosis [55]. Frequencies of individual symptoms at the final observation point were shown in Tables 1.2 and 1.6

Table 1.6 Initial symptoms and duration from symptom onset to diagnosis

Symptoms	Kim[a]	Ideguchi[b]		
	Korea	Japan		
	1988	2011		
	$n=410$	$n=412$		
	(%)	(%)	Duration to diagnosis (years)	Final (%)[c]
Oral aphtha	80.5	70.4	−7.5 ± 10.2	99.5
Genital ulcer	7.3	16.0	−1.5 ± 5.4	72.6
Skin lesions	7.1	23.5	−1.7 ± 5.7	88.1
Eye lesions	3.2	13.6	−1.1 ± 4.6	64.6
Arthritis	1.9	7.5	1.3 ± 8.0	48.1
Epididymitis		0.0	−0.1 ± 1.2	6.0
GI involvement		1.5	1.9 ± 5.0	10.4
CNS involvement		0.7	4.0 ± 7.1	13.1
Vascular involvement		1.2	2.2 ± 8.4	6.3
Any manifestations			−8.6 ± 10.2	

In both studies, the diagnosis was made by the Japan criteria
[a]The first single symptom is considered as an initial symptom [62]
[b]All symptoms which simultaneously appeared at the onset are considered as initial symptoms [55]
[c]Cumulative frequency at the final point of observation

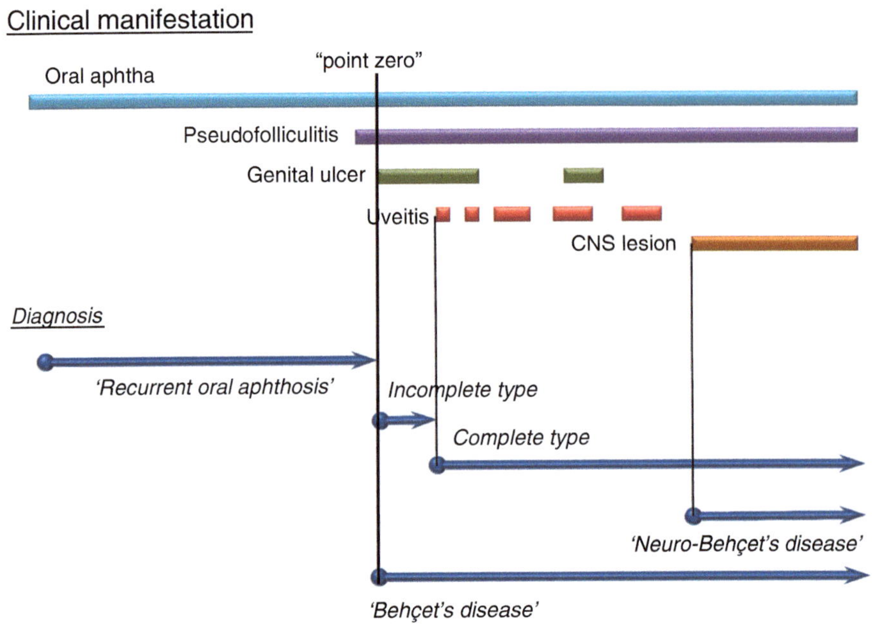

Fig. 1.2 Clinical course of a putative patient
The *upper part* shows appearance of each symptom, whereas the corresponding clinical diagnoses at the individual points are shown in the *lower part*, according to classification of the Japan revised criteria

symptoms. On the contrary, gastrointestinal, CNS, and large vessel lesions develop as late complications after the diagnosis is established, though they can precede major symptoms in a minority of patients.

Clinical phenotype is not consistent during the clinical course in individual patients. Rather, it can evolve. Figure 1.2 shows a clinical course in a putative male patient. He had been suffering from recurrent oral aphthosis for more than 10 years until he first visited a clinic when he presented with pseudofolliculitis and genital ulcers. He is not exceptional. Most patients do not see physicians due to oral aphtha alone because they have no idea that oral aphtha is the first sign of systemic disease. At this point, he was diagnosed with BD, incomplete type, according to the classification of the Japan criteria [55]. A year later, he repeatedly experienced ocular attacks due to uveitis, leading to the diagnosis of BD, complete type [55]. The diagnosis was further revised as neuro-BD when neurological involvement developed 5 years later [55]. This is a putative patient, but the clinical course can be realistic except therapeutic interventions are not considered.

Individual BD patients may have more complicated and heterogeneous clinical courses in the real world. A long-term cohort study from Turkey has shown that mucocutaneous symptoms and arthritis are subsided during the clinical course in

Table 1.7 Chronological changes of mucocutaneous and articular manifestations

Manifestations	Initial visit (%)	Final visit (%)
Oral ulceration	100	63.7
Genital ulceration	89.9	26.1
Erythema nodosum	64.6	25.5
Papulopustular lesions	84.3	35.7
Arthritis	40.6	9.9
Fulfillment of O'Duffy criteria	100	27.2

Symptoms were confirmed in outpatient clinics or over telephone

many patients (Table 1.7) [71]. In a long-term cohort study in which O'Duffy criteria for the diagnosis were used as inclusion criteria, only 27 % of the patients (94/345) would have fulfilled the criteria if one considered the disease manifestations only within the latest year [71]. Thus, it is impossible to make the diagnosis correctly based on clinical findings in a single time point. It is reasonable that all of the clinical manifestations along the course are taken into account when making the diagnosis or classification of BD according to a set of criteria.

1.5 Prognosis

BD significantly increases morbidity and mortality [59, 71]. The leading cause of morbidity in BD is ocular involvement with the potential threat of blindness. The details will be discussed in Sect. 4.5. Table 1.8 compares causes of death in BD patients between two cohort studies from Turkey and France. Both show very similar data. Most of patients who died due to BD were male at younger than 50 years old. Young aged onset and frequent flares were also predisposing factors to BD-related death.

Among the disease subtypes, large vascular involvement is the most common cause of death in patients with BD [59, 71]. A number of studies also have revealed that arterial lesions, especially pulmonary arterial aneurysms (PAA), are associated with fatal events [60, 72–75]. Yacizi et al. have conducted three consecutive cohort studies in a single institute from Turkey [72, 73, 75]. The studies have shown that prognosis in patients with PAA was improved by introduction of aggressive immunosuppressive therapies. However, even in the latest report in 2012, 9 of 34 patients (26 %) died for 3.6 ± 5.2 years of observation period. Besides PAA, aortic aneurysms, Budd-Chiari syndrome, and superior and/or inferior vena cava syndrome can be fatal. Details are described in Chap. 5. CNS involvement, particularly chronic progressive type, is another cause of death in BD patients [59, 71, 76] (see Chap. 6). Of malignancies, several studies have shown association between myelodysplastic

Table 1.8 Major causes of death in BD patients from two cohort studies

		Kural-Seyahi[a]		Saadoun[a]	
		Turkey		France	
		2003		2010	
All patients		428		817	
	M/F	286	142	541	276
	Rate of male	66.8 %		66.2 %	
	Observation (years)	15–23		7.7	
Died patients		42	9.8 %	41	5.0 %
	Age of death (years)	40.4±16.7		34.6±11.5	
	M/F	39	3	38	3
	Rate of male	92.9 %		92.7 %	
Causes of death					
Large vessel involvement		20	47.6 %	18	43.9 %
	PAA[b]	9	21.4 %	3	7.3 %
	Aortic aneurysm	1	2.4 %	4	9.8 %
	Ischemic heart disease	3	7.1 %	3	7.3 %
	Budd-Chiari syndrome	3	7.1 %	4	9.8 %
	SVC/IVC syndrome	4	9.5 %		
	Pulmonary embolism			3	7.3 %
CNS		5	11.9 %	5	12.2 %
Cancer and malignancy		4	9.5 %	6	14.6 %
Infection				5	12.2 %

[a]References are [59] and [71]
[b]*PAA* pulmonary artery aneurysm

syndrome and BD, especially intestinal BD [77–79]. Like other autoimmune diseases and vasculitis syndromes, immunosuppression-related infection can be another cause of death.

1.6 New Therapeutic Options – Biologics and Others

The main therapeutic goal in BD is to induce and maintain remission and prevent irreversible damage from eye and organ involvement. To improve patient's quality of life is another goal. Because clinical manifestations of BD patients show heterogeneous symptoms with diverse severity, it is impossible to determine a single management strategy for all patients. Different therapeutic approaches are necessary for individual symptoms, though some of them are shared [3, 4]. EULAR developed nine recommendations for different aspects of BD (Table 1.9) [3]. It is a rule that therapy is focused on the most serious symptom.

Table 1.9 Nine recommendations by EULAR

No.	Recommendation	Category of evidence	Strength of recommendation
1.	Any patient with BD and inflammatory eye disease affecting the posterior segment should be on a treatment regime that includes azathioprine and systemic corticosteroids	Ib	A/D
2.	If the patient has severe eye disease defined as .2 lines of drop in visual acuity on a 10/10 scale and/or retinal disease (retinal vasculitis or macular involvement), it is recommended that either cyclosporine A or infliximab be used in combination with azathioprine and corticosteroids; alternatively IFNα with or without corticosteroids could be used instead	Ib/Iib	C/D
3.	There is no firm evidence to guide the management of major vessel disease in BD. For the management of acute deep vein thrombosis in BD immunosuppressive agents such as corticosteroids, azathioprine, cyclophosphamide, or cyclosporine A are recommended. For the management of pulmonary and peripheral arterial aneurysms, cyclophosphamide and corticosteroids are recommended	III	C
4.	Similarly there are no controlled data on, or evidence of benefit from uncontrolled experience with anticoagulants, antiplatelet, or antifibrinolytic agents in the management of deep vein thrombosis or for the use of anticoagulation for the arterial lesions of BD	IV	D
5.	There is no evidence-based treatment that can be recommended for the management of gastrointestinal involvement of BD. Agents such as sulfasalazine, corticosteroids, azathioprine, TNFα antagonists, and thalidomide should be tried first before surgery, except in emergencies	III	C
6.	In most patients with BD, arthritis can be managed with colchicine	Ib	A
7.	There are no controlled data to guide the management of CNS involvement in BD. For parenchymal involvement agents, to be tried may include corticosteroids, IFNα, azathioprine, cyclophosphamide, methotrexate, and TNFα antagonists. For dural sinus thrombosis, corticosteroids are recommended	III	C
8.	Cyclosporine A should not be used in BD patients with central nervous system involvement unless necessary for intraocular inflammation	III	C/D

(continued)

Table 1.9 (continued)

No.	Recommendation	Category of evidence	Strength of recommendation
9.	The decision to treat skin and mucosa involvement will depend on the perceived severity by the doctor and the patient. Mucocutaneous involvement should be treated according to the dominant or codominant lesions present	Ib	A/C
	Topical measures (i.e., local corticosteroids) should be the first line of treatment for isolated oral and genital ulcers		
	Acne-like lesions are usually of cosmetic concern only. Thus, topical measures as used in acne vulgaris are sufficient		
	Colchicine should be preferred when the dominant lesion is erythema nodosum		
	Leg ulcers in BD might have different causes. Treatment should be planned accordingly		
	Azathioprine, IFNα, and TNFα antagonists may be considered in resistant cases		

Reference [3] is modified

Over the last decade, a number of studies have shown clinical efficacy of TNF inhibitors for uveitis, gastrointestinal involvement, and CNS lesions in patients with BD [4, 16, 17, 19, 20, 23, 80, 81]. Infliximab and adalimumab have been approved for treatment of refractory uveitis since 2007 and for gastrointestinal involvement since 2013 in Japan, respectively. A post-marketing survey of infliximab revealed that the response rate was reported as 90 % at one year in patients with refractory uveitis. Infliximab potently suppresses ocular attacks, leading to improvement of visual acuity in most of patients, though discontinuation of the agent is commonly associated with relapsing ocular attacks [16, 17, 19]. In addition, the clinical trial for intestinal, CNS, and vascular lesions in BD patients is now underway in Japan. It is very promising.

Recently, an open-label pilot study of anti-IL-1 mAb, gevokizumab showed rapid and sustained reduction of ocular inflammation in BD patients without major adverse events [82]. Favorable outcomes were also reported in clinical trials for anti-CD20 mAb, rituximab for uveitis [83]. Sporadic case reports have shown beneficial effects of anti-IL-6 receptor mAb, tocilizumab, on neuro-BD [84]. We need to accumulate further data until clinical application of these agents can be applied to serious form of manifestations in BD patients. Alternatively, an effect of phosphodiesterase (PDE) inhibitor on oral aphthae was reported [85].

1.7 Summary

This chapter summaries general overviews in clinical aspects of BD. It would be helpful for the readers to understand current topics discussed in the following chapters.

References

1. Behçet H. Uber rezidivierende, aphthose, dürch ein Virus versachte Geshwure am Munde, am Auge und an den Genitalien. Dermatoogishche Wochenschrift. 1937;36:1152–557.
2. Sakane T, Takeno M, Suzuki N, Inaba G. Behcet's disease. N Engl J Med. 1999;341(17):1284–91. doi:10.1056/nejm199910213411707.
3. Hatemi G, Silman A, Bang D, Bodaghi B, Chamberlain AM, Gul A, Houman MH, Kotter I, Olivieri I, Salvarani C, Sfikakis PP, Siva A, Stanford MR, Stubiger N, Yurdakul S, Yazici H, Committee EE. EULAR recommendations for the management of Behcet disease. Ann Rheum Dis. 2008;67(12):1656–62. doi:10.1136/ard.2007.080432.
4. Hatemi G, Silman A, Bang D, Bodaghi B, Chamberlain AM, Gul A, Houman MH, Kotter I, Olivieri I, Salvarani C, Sfikakis PP, Siva A, Stanford MR, Stubiger N, Yurdakul S, Yazici H. Management of Behcet disease: a systematic literature review for the European League Against Rheumatism evidence-based recommendations for the management of Behcet disease. Ann Rheum Dis. 2009;68(10):1528–34. doi:10.1136/ard.2008.087957.
5. Sfikakis PP, Markomichelakis N, Alpsoy E, Assaad-Khalil S, Bodaghi B, Gul A, Ohno S, Pipitone N, Schirmer M, Stanford M, Wechsler B, Zouboulis C, Kaklamanis P, Yazici H. Anti-TNF therapy in the management of Behcet's disease – review and basis for recommendations. Rheumatology. 2007;46(5):736–41. doi:10.1093/rheumatology/kem034.
6. Kalra S, Silman A, Akman-Demir G, Bohlega S, Borhani-Haghighi A, Constantinescu CS, Houman H, Mahr A, Salvarani C, Sfikakis PP, Siva A, Al-Araji A. Diagnosis and management of Neuro-Behcet's disease: international consensus recommendations. J Neurol. 2013. doi:10.1007/s00415-013-7209-3.
7. Levy-Clarke G, Jabs DA, Read RW, Rosenbaum JT, Vitale A, Van Gelder RN. Expert panel recommendations for the use of anti-tumor necrosis factor biologic agents in patients with ocular inflammatory disorders. Ophthalmology. 2014;121(3):785–796.e783. doi:10.1016/j.ophtha.2013.09.048.
8. Jennette JC, Falk RJ, Bacon PA, Basu N, Cid MC, Ferrario F, Flores-Suarez LF, Gross WL, Guillevin L, Hagen EC, Hoffman GS, Jayne DR, Kallenberg CG, Lamprecht P, Langford CA, Luqmani RA, Mahr AD, Matteson EL, Merkel PA, Ozen S, Pusey CD, Rasmussen N, Rees AJ, Scott DG, Specks U, Stone JH, Takahashi K, Watts RA. 2012 revised international Chapel Hill consensus conference nomenclature of vasculitides. Arthritis Rheum. 2013;65(1):1–11. doi:10.1002/art.37715.
9. Mizuki N, Meguro A, Ota M, Ohno S, Shiota T, Kawagoe T, Ito N, Kera J, Okada E, Yatsu K, Song YW, Lee EB, Kitaichi N, Namba K, Horie Y, Takeno M, Sugita S, Mochizuki M, Bahram S, Ishigatsubo Y, Inoko H. Genome-wide association studies identify IL23R-IL12RB2 and IL10 as Behcet's disease susceptibility loci. Nat Genet. 2010;42(8):703–6. doi:10.1038/ng.624.
10. Remmers EF, Cosan F, Kirino Y, Ombrello MJ, Abaci N, Satorius C, Le JM, Yang B, Korman BD, Cakiris A, Aglar O, Emrence Z, Azakli H, Ustek D, Tugal-Tutkun I, Akman-Demir G, Chen W, Amos CI, Dizon MB, Kose AA, Azizlerli G, Erer B, Brand OJ, Kaklamani VG, Kaklamanis P, Ben-Chetrit E, Stanford M, Fortune F, Ghabra M, Ollier WE, Cho YH, Bang D, O'Shea J,

Wallace GR, Gadina M, Kastner DL, Gul A. Genome-wide association study identifies variants in the MHC class I, IL10, and IL23R-IL12RB2 regions associated with Behcet's disease. Nat Genet. 2010;42(8):698–702. doi:10.1038/ng.625.

11. Kirino Y, Bertsias G, Ishigatsubo Y, Mizuki N, Tugal-Tutkun I, Seyahi E, Ozyazgan Y, Sacli FS, Erer B, Inoko H, Emrence Z, Cakar A, Abaci N, Ustek D, Satorius C, Ueda A, Takeno M, Kim Y, Wood GM, Ombrello MJ, Meguro A, Gul A, Remmers EF, Kastner DL. Genome-wide association analysis identifies new susceptibility loci for Behcet's disease and epistasis between HLA-B*51 and ERAP1. Nat Genet. 2013;45(2):202–7. doi:10.1038/ng.2520.
12. Kirino Y, Zhou Q, Ishigatsubo Y, Mizuki N, Tugal-Tutkun I, Seyahi E, Ozyazgan Y, Ugurlu S, Erer B, Abaci N, Ustek D, Meguro A, Ueda A, Takeno M, Inoko H, Ombrello MJ, Satorius CL, Maskeri B, Mullikin JC, Sun HW, Gutierrez-Cruz G, Kim Y, Wilson AF, Kastner DL, Gul A, Remmers EF. Targeted resequencing implicates the familial Mediterranean fever gene MEFV and the toll-like receptor 4 gene TLR4 in Behcet disease. Proc Natl Acad Sci U S A. 2013;110(20):8134–9. doi:10.1073/pnas.1306352110.
13. Hou S, Yang Z, Du L, Jiang Z, Shu Q, Chen Y, Li F, Zhou Q, Ohno S, Chen R, Kijlstra A, Rosenbaum JT, Yang P. Identification of a susceptibility locus in STAT4 for Behcet's disease in Han Chinese in a genome-wide association study. Arthritis Rheum. 2012;64(12):4104–13. doi:10.1002/art.37708.
14. Hou S, Xiao X, Li F, Jiang Z, Kijlstra A, Yang P. Two-stage association study in Chinese Han identifies two independent associations in CCR1/CCR3 locus as candidate for Behcet's disease susceptibility. Hum Genet. 2012;131(12):1841–50. doi:10.1007/s00439-012-1200-4.
15. Xavier JM, Shahram F, Davatchi F, Rosa A, Crespo J, Abdollahi BS, Nadji A, Jesus G, Barcelos F, Patto JV, Shafiee NM, Ghaderibarim F, Oliveira SA. Association study of IL10 and IL23R-IL12RB2 in Iranian patients with Behcet's disease. Arthritis Rheum. 2012;64(8):2761–72. doi:10.1002/art.34437.
16. Ohno S, Nakamura S, Hori S, Shimakawa M, Kawashima H, Mochizuki M, Sugita S, Ueno S, Yoshizaki K, Inaba G. Efficacy, safety, and pharmacokinetics of multiple administration of infliximab in Behcet's disease with refractory uveoretinitis. J Rheumatol. 2004;31(7):1362–8.
17. Arida A, Fragiadaki K, Giavri E, Sfikakis PP. Anti-TNF agents for Behcet's disease: analysis of published data on 369 patients. Semin Arthritis Rheum. 2011;41(1):61–70. doi:10.1016/j.semarthrit.2010.09.002.
18. Okada AA, Goto H, Ohno S, Mochizuki M. Multicenter study of infliximab for refractory uveoretinitis in Behcet disease. Arch Ophthalmol. 2012;130(5):592–8. doi:10.1001/archophthalmol.2011.2698.
19. Calvo-Rio V, Blanco R, Beltran E, Sanchez-Burson J, Mesquida M, Adan A, Hernandez MV, Hernandez Garfella M, Valls Pascual E, Martinez-Costa L, Sellas-Fernandez A, Cordero Coma M, Diaz-Llopis M, Gallego R, Salom D, Garcia Serrano JL, Ortego N, Herreras JM, Fonollosa A, Garcia-Aparicio AM, Maiz O, Blanco A, Torre I, Fernandez-Espartero C, Jovani V, Peiteado-Lopez D, Pato E, Cruz J, Fernandez-Cid C, Aurrecoechea E, Garcia M, Caracuel MA, Montilla C, Atanes A, Hernandez FF, Insua S, Gonzalez-Suarez S, Sanchez-Andrade A, Gamero F, Linares L, Romero-Bueno F, Garcia AJ, Almodovar R, Minguez E, Carrasco Cubero C, Olive A, Vazquez J, Ruiz Moreno O, Jimenez-Zorzo F, Manero J, Munoz Fernandez S, Rueda-Gotor J, Gonzalez-Gay MA. Anti-TNF-alpha therapy in patients with refractory uveitis due to Behcet's disease: a 1-year follow-up study of 124 patients. Rheumatology. 2014. doi:10.1093/rheumatology/keu266.
20. Iwata S, Saito K, Yamaoka K, Tsujimura S, Nawata M, Suzuki K, Tanaka Y. Effects of anti-TNF-alpha antibody infliximab in refractory entero-Behcet's disease. Rheumatology. 2009;48(8):1012–13. doi:10.1093/rheumatology/kep126.
21. Hisamatsu T, Ueno F, Matsumoto T, Kobayashi K, Koganei K, Kunisaki R, Hirai F, Nagahori M, Matsushita M, Kobayashi K, Kishimoto M, Takeno M, Tanaka M, Inoue N, Hibi T. The 2nd edition of consensus statements for the diagnosis and management of intestinal Behcet's disease: indication of anti-TNFalpha monoclonal antibodies. J Gastroenterol. 2014;49(1):156–62. doi:10.1007/s00535-013-0872-4.

22. Ideguchi H, Suda A, Takeno M, Miyagi R, Ueda A, Ohno S, Ishigatsubo Y. Gastrointestinal manifestations of Behcet's disease in Japan: a study of 43 patients. Rheumatol Int. 2014;34(6):851–6. doi:10.1007/s00296-013-2838-5.
23. Kikuchi H, Aramaki K, Hirohata S. Effect of infliximab in progressive neuro-Behcet's syndrome. J Neurol Sci. 2008;272(1–2):99–105. doi:10.1016/j.jns.2008.05.002.
24. Silvestri E, Emmi G, Prisco D. Anti-TNF-alpha agents in vascular Behcet's disease. Expert Rev Cardiovasc Ther. 2014;12(4):415–16. doi:10.1586/14779072.2014.896198.
25. Adler S, Baumgartner I, Villiger PM. Behcet's disease: successful treatment with infliximab in 7 patients with severe vascular manifestations. A retrospective analysis. Arthritis Care Res. 2012;64(4):607–11. doi:10.1002/acr.21557.
26. Yurdakul S, Yazici H. Behcet's syndrome. Best Pract Res Clin Rheumatol. 2008;22(5):793–809. doi:10.1016/j.berh.2008.08.005.
27. Yurdakul S, Gunaydin I, Tuzun Y, Tankurt N, Pazarli H, Ozyazgan Y, Yazici H. The prevalence of Behcet's syndrome in a rural area in northern Turkey. J Rheumatol. 1988;15(5):820–2.
28. Idil A, Gurler A, Boyvat A, Caliskan D, Ozdemir O, Isik A, Tuncbilek A, Kocyigit P, Calikoglu E. The prevalence of Behcet's disease above the age of 10 years. The results of a pilot study conducted at the Park Primary Health Care Center in Ankara, Turkey. Ophthalmic Epidemiol. 2002;9(5):325–31.
29. Azizlerli G, Kose AA, Sarica R, Gul A, Tutkun IT, Kulac M, Tunc R, Urgancioglu M, Disci R. Prevalence of Behcet's disease in Istanbul, Turkey. Int J Dermatol. 2003;42(10):803–6.
30. Cakir N, Dervis E, Benian O, Pamuk ON, Sonmezates N, Rahimoglu R, Tuna S, Cetin T, Sarikaya Y. Prevalence of Behcet's disease in rural western Turkey: a preliminary report. Clin Exp Rheumatol. 2004;22(4 Suppl 34):S53–5.
31. Yamamoto S, Toyokawa H, Matsubara J, et al. A nation wide survey of Behçet's disease in Japan. Jpn J Ophthalmol. 1974;18:282–90.
32. Nakae KMF, Hashimoto T, Inaba G, Mochizuki M, Sakane T. Recent epidemiological features of Behcet's disease in Japan. In: Godeau P, Wechsler B, editors. Behcet's disease. Amsterdam: Excerpta Medica; 1993. p. 145–51.
33. Mahr A, Belarbi L, Wechsler B, Jeanneret D, Dhote R, Fain O, Lhote F, Ramanoelina J, Coste J, Guillevin L. Population-based prevalence study of Behcet's disease: differences by ethnic origin and low variation by age at immigration. Arthritis Rheum. 2008;58(12):3951–9. doi:10.1002/art.24149.
34. Davatchi F, Shahram F, Chams-Davatchi C, Shams H, Nadji A, Akhlaghi M, Faezi T, Ghodsi Z, Faridar A, Ashofteh F, Sadeghi Abdollahi B. Behcet's disease: from East to West. Clin Rheumatol. 2010;29(8):823–33. doi:10.1007/s10067-010-1430-6.
35. Al-Rawi ZS, Neda AH. Prevalence of Behcet's disease among Iraqis. Adv Exp Med Biol. 2003;528:37–41. doi:10.1007/0-306-48382-3_6.
36. Gonzalez-Gay MA, Garcia-Porrua C, Branas F, Lopez-Lazaro L, Olivieri I. Epidemiologic and clinical aspects of Behcet's disease in a defined area of Northwestern Spain, 1988–1997. J Rheumatol. 2000;27(3):703–7.
37. Grana J, Sanchez-Meizoso MO, Galdo F. Epidemiological aspects of Behcet's disease in Galicia. J Rheumatol. 2001;28(11):2565–6.
38. Salvarani C, Pipitone N, Catanoso MG, Cimino L, Tumiati B, Macchioni P, Bajocchi G, Olivieri I, Boiardi L. Epidemiology and clinical course of Behcet's disease in the Reggio Emilia area of Northern Italy: a seventeen-year population-based study. Arthritis Rheum. 2007;57(1):171–8. doi:10.1002/art.22500.
39. Zouboulis CC, Kotter I, Djawari D, Kirch W, Kohl PK, Ochsendorf FR, Keitel W, Stadler R, Wollina U, Proksch E, Sohnchen R, Weber H, Gollnick HP, Holzle E, Fritz K, Licht T, Orfanos CE. Epidemiological features of Adamantiades-Behcet's disease in Germany and in Europe. Yonsei Med J. 1997;38(6):411–22.
40. Papoutsis NG, Abdel-Naser MB, Altenburg A, Orawa H, Kotter I, Krause L, Pleyer U, Djawari D, Stadler R, Wollina U, Kohl PK, Gollnick HP, Kirch W, Ochsendorf FR, Keitel W, Martus P, Zouboulis CC. Prevalence of Adamantiades-Behcet's disease in Germany and the municipality of Berlin: results of a nationwide survey. Clin Exp Rheumatol. 2006;24(5 Suppl 42):S125.

41. Chamberlain MA. Behcet's syndrome in 32 patients in Yorkshire. Ann Rheum Dis. 1977;36(6):491–9.
42. Jankowski J, Crombie I, Jankowski R. Behcet's syndrome in Scotland. Postgrad Med J. 1992;68(801):566–70.
43. Ek L, Hedfors E. Behcet's disease: a review and a report of 12 cases from Sweden. Acta Derm Venereol. 1993;73(4):251–4.
44. Mok CC, Cheung TC, Ho CT, Lee KW, Lau CS, Wong RW. Behcet's disease in southern Chinese patients. J Rheumatol. 2002;29(8):1689–93.
45. Chen YC, Chang HW. Clinical characteristics of Behcet's disease in southern Taiwan. J Microbiol Immunol Infect=Wei mian yu gan ran za zhi. 2001;34(3):207–10.
46. O'Duffy JD. Summary of international symposium on Behcet's disease. Istanbul, September 29–30, 1977. J Rheumatol. 1978;5(2):229–33.
47. Verity DH, Marr JE, Ohno S, Wallace GR, Stanford MR. Behcet's disease, the Silk Road and HLA-B51: historical and geographical perspectives. Tissue Antigens. 1999;54(3):213–20.
48. Jaber L, Milo G, Halpern GJ, Krause I, Weinberger A. Prevalence of Behcet's disease in an Arab community in Israel. Ann Rheum Dis. 2002;61(4):365–6.
49. Krause I, Yankevich A, Fraser A, Rosner I, Mader R, Zisman D, Boulman N, Rozenbaum M, Weinberger A. Prevalence and clinical aspects of Behcet's disease in the north of Israel. Clin Rheumatol. 2007;26(4):555–60. doi:10.1007/s10067-006-0349-4.
50. Hirohata T, Kuratsune M, Nomura A, Jimi S. Prevalence of Behcet's syndrome in Hawaii. With particular reference to the comparison of the Japanese in Hawaii and Japan. Hawaii Med J. 1975;34(7):244–6.
51. Gul A, Inanc M, Ocal L, Aral O, Konice M. Familial aggregation of Behcet's disease in Turkey. Ann Rheum Dis. 2000;59(8):622–5.
52. Hayasaka S, Kurome H, Noda S. HLA antigens in a Japanese family with Behcet's disease. Graefe's Arch Clin Exp Ophthalmol=Albrecht von Graefes Archiv fur klinische und experimentelle Ophthalmologie. 1994;232(10):589–90.
53. Kone-Paut I, Geisler I, Wechsler B, Ozen S, Ozdogan H, Rozenbaum M, Touitou I. Familial aggregation in Behcet's disease: high frequency in siblings and parents of pediatric probands. J Pediatr. 1999;135(1):89–93.
54. Taylor SR, Singh J, Menezo V, Wakefield D, McCluskey P, Lightman S. Behcet disease: visual prognosis and factors influencing the development of visual loss. Am J Ophthalmol. 2011;152(6):1059–66. doi:10.1016/j.ajo.2011.05.032.
55. Ideguchi H, Suda A, Takeno M, Ueda A, Ohno S, Ishigatsubo Y. Behcet disease: evolution of clinical manifestations. Medicine. 2011;90(2):125–32. doi:10.1097/MD.0b013e318211bf28.
56. Ideguchi H, Suda A, Takeno M, Kirino Y, Ihata A, Ueda A, Ohno S, Baba Y, Kuroiwa Y, Ishigatsubo Y. Neurological manifestations of Behcet's disease in Japan: a study of 54 patients. J Neurol. 2010;257(6):1012–20. doi:10.1007/s00415-010-5454-2.
57. Hirohata S, Kikuchi H, Sawada T, Nagafuchi H, Kuwana M, Takeno M, Ishigatsubo Y. Clinical characteristics of neuro-Behcet's disease in Japan: a multicenter retrospective analysis. Mod Rheumatol/Jpn Rheum Assoc. 2012;22(3):405–13. doi:10.1007/s10165-011-0533-5.
58. Noel N, Bernard R, Wechsler B, Resche-Rigon M, Depaz R, Boutin DL, Piette JC, Drier A, Dormont D, Cacoub P, Saadoun D. Long-term outcome of neuro-Behcet's disease. Arthritis Rheum. 2014;66(5):1306–14. doi:10.1002/art.38351.
59. Saadoun D, Wechsler B, Desseaux K, Le Thi Huong D, Amoura Z, Resche-Rigon M, Cacoub P. Mortality in Behcet's disease. Arthritis Rheum. 2010;62(9):2806–12. doi:10.1002/art.27568.
60. Saadoun D, Asli B, Wechsler B, Houman H, Geri G, Desseaux K, Piette JC, du Huong LT, Amoura Z, Salem TB, Cluzel P, Koskas F, Resche-Rigon M, Cacoub P. Long-term outcome of arterial lesions in Behcet disease: a series of 101 patients. Medicine. 2012;91(1):18–24. doi:10.1097/MD.0b013e3182428126.
61. Yurdakul S, Yazici Y. (2010) Epidemiology of Behcet's syndrome and regional differences in disease expression. Behcet's Syndrome (Yazici Y and Yazici H):35–52.
62. Kim HJ, Bang D, Lee SH, Yang DS, Kim DH, Lee KH, Lee S, Kim HB, Hong WP. Behcet's syndrome in Korea: a look at the clinical picture. Yonsei Med J. 1988;29(1):72–8.

63. Criteria for diagnosis of Behcet's disease. International Study Group for Behcet's Disease (1990). Lancet 335 (8697):1078–1080.
64. Lee S. Diagnostic criteria of Behcet's disease: problems and suggestions. Yonsei Med J. 1997;38(6):365–9.
65. Faezi ST, Paragomi P, Shahram F, Shams H, Shams-Davatchi C, Ghodsi Z, Nadji A, Akhlaghi M, Davatchi F. Clinical features of Behcet's disease in patients without oral aphthosis. Mod Rheumatol/Jpn Rheum Assoc. 2014;24(4):637–9. doi:10.3109/14397595.2013.844400.
66. Dilsen N, Konice M, Aral O, Ocal L, Inanc M, Gul A. Comparative study of the skin pathergy test with blunt and sharp needles in Behcet's disease: confirmed specificity but decreased sensitivity with sharp needles. Ann Rheum Dis. 1993;52(11):823–5.
67. Davatchi F, Chams-Davatchi C, Ghodsi Z, Shahram F, Nadji A, Shams H, Akhlaghi M, Larimi R, Sadeghi-Abdolahi B. Diagnostic value of pathergy test in Behcet's disease according to the change of incidence over the time. Clin Rheumatol. 2011;30(9):1151–5. doi:10.1007/s10067-011-1694-5.
68. Davatchi F, Sadeghi Abdollahi B, Chams-Davatchi C, Shahram F, Ghodsi Z, Nadji A, Akhlaghi M, Faezi T, Shams H, Larimi R, Ashofteh F. Impact of the positive pathergy test on the performance of classification/diagnosis criteria for Behcet's disease. Mod Rheumatol/Jpn Rheum Assoc. 2013;23(1):125–32. doi:10.1007/s10165-012-0626-9.
69. Davatchi F, Abdollahi BS, Chams-Davatchi C, Shahram F, Nadji A, Shams H, Faezi T, Akhlaghi M, Ashofteh F, Mataji M, Moradi K, Mohtasham N. Validation of the revised International Criteria for Behcet's Disease (ICBD) in Iran. Clin Rheumatol. 2013. doi:10.1007/s10067-013-2411-3.
70. International Team for the Revision of the International Criteria for Behcet's D. The International Criteria for Behcet's Disease (ICBD): a collaborative study of 27 countries on the sensitivity and specificity of the new criteria. J Eur Acad Dermatol Venereol. 2014;28(3):338–47. doi:10.1111/jdv.12107.
71. Kural-Seyahi E, Fresko I, Seyahi N, Ozyazgan Y, Mat C, Hamuryudan V, Yurdakul S, Yazici H. The long-term mortality and morbidity of Behcet syndrome: a 2-decade outcome survey of 387 patients followed at a dedicated center. Medicine. 2003;82(1):60–76.
72. Hamuryudan V, Yurdakul S, Moral F, Numan F, Tuzun H, Tuzuner N, Mat C, Tuzun Y, Ozyazgan Y, Yazici H. Pulmonary arterial aneurysms in Behcet's syndrome: a report of 24 cases. Br J Rheumatol. 1994;33(1):48–51.
73. Hamuryudan V, Er T, Seyahi E, Akman C, Tuzun H, Fresko I, Yurdakul S, Numan F, Yazici H. Pulmonary artery aneurysms in Behcet syndrome. Am J Med. 2004;117(11):867–70. doi:10.1016/j.amjmed.2004.05.027.
74. Uzun O, Akpolat T, Erkan L. Pulmonary vasculitis in behcet disease: a cumulative analysis. Chest. 2005;127(6):2243–53. doi:10.1378/chest.127.6.2243.
75. Seyahi E, Melikoglu M, Akman C, Hamuryudan V, Ozer H, Hatemi G, Yurdakul S, Tuzun H, Oz B, Yazici H. Pulmonary artery involvement and associated lung disease in Behcet disease: a series of 47 patients. Medicine. 2012;91(1):35–48. doi:10.1097/MD.0b013e318242ff37.
76. Noel N, Bernard R, Wechsler B, Resche-Rigon M, Depaz R, Le Thi Huong Boutin D, Piette J-C, Drier A, Dormont D, Cacoub P, Saadoun D. Long-term outcome of neuro-Behçet's disease. Arthritis Rheumatol. 2014;66(5):1306–14. doi:10.1002/art.38351.
77. Ahn JK, Oh JM, Lee J, Koh EM, Cha HS. Behcet's disease associated with malignancy in Korea: a single center experience. Rheumatol Int. 2010;30(6):831–5. doi:10.1007/s00296-009-1319-3.
78. Tada Y, Koarada S, Haruta Y, Mitamura M, Ohta A, Nagasawa K. The association of Behcet's disease with myelodysplastic syndrome in Japan: a review of the literature. Clin Exp Rheumatol. 2006;24(5 Suppl 42):S115–19.
79. Lin Y, Li G, Zheng W, Tian X, Zhang F. Behcet's disease associated with malignancy: a report of 41 Chinese cases. Int J Rheum Dis. 2014;17(4):459–65. doi:10.1111/1756-185x.12269.
80. Saleh Z, Arayssi T. Update on the therapy of Behcet disease. Ther Adv Chronic Dis. 2014;5(3):112–34. doi:10.1177/2040622314523062.
81. Comarmond C, Wechsler B, Bodaghi B, Cacoub P, Saadoun D. Biotherapies in Behcet's disease. Autoimmun Rev. 2014;13(7):762–9. doi:10.1016/j.autrev.2014.01.056.

82. Gul A, Tugal-Tutkun I, Dinarello CA, Reznikov L, Esen BA, Mirza A, Scannon P, Solinger A. Interleukin-1beta-regulating antibody XOMA 052 (gevokizumab) in the treatment of acute exacerbations of resistant uveitis of Behcet's disease: an open-label pilot study. Ann Rheum Dis. 2012;71(4):563–6. doi:10.1136/annrheumdis-2011-155143.
83. Davatchi F, Shams H, Rezaipoor M, Sadeghi-Abdollahi B, Shahram F, Nadji A, Chams-Davatchi C, Akhlaghi M, Faezi T, Naderi N. Rituximab in intractable ocular lesions of Behcet's disease; randomized single-blind control study (pilot study). Int J Rheum Dis. 2010;13(3):246–52. doi:10.1111/j.1756-185X.2010.01546.x.
84. Hirano T, Ohguro N, Hohki S, Hagihara K, Shima Y, Narazaki M, Ogata A, Yoshizaki K, Kumanogoh A, Kishimoto T, Tanaka T. A case of Behcet's disease treated with a humanized anti-interleukin-6 receptor antibody, tocilizumab. Mod Rheumatol/Jpn Rheum Assoc. 2012;22(2):298–302. doi:10.1007/s10165-011-0497-5.
85. Hatemi G, et al. (2013) ACR Annual Meeting. Abstract 761.

Chapter 2
The Immunopathology of Behçet's Disease

Noboru Suzuki and Jun Shimizu

Abstract Aberrant immune functions including but not restricted to skewed T cell responses and intrinsic activation of B lymphocytes contributed to the development of Behçet's disease (BD). Recently, we found that Th17 cells, a new helper T (Th) cell subset which produces IL17 family cytokines, increased in patients with BD. Precise analyses disclosed that Th1/Th17 cells which harbor both phenotypes of IFNgamma-producing cells and that of IL17-producing cells simultaneously increased significantly in patients with BD.

We found that macrophages/monocytes regulated Th cell differentiation through a heat-shock protein (HSP) in both systemic immune system and local inflammatory lesions in patients with BD. Here, we summarize current findings on Th cell differentiation, antigen-presenting cell (APC) activation, and their contribution to the pathogenesis of BD, especially in view of IL12/IL23 family cytokine production and pattern recognition receptor (PRR) function of macrophages/monocytes.

Keywords Th1 cells • Th17 cells • IFNgamma-producing Th17 cells • IL12/IL23 family cytokines • Innate immunity • Pattern recognition receptor

2.1 Introduction

Behçet's disease (BD) is a systemic inflammatory disease, characterized by recurrent signs and symptoms of oral aphthosis, genital ulcers, skin lesions, and uveitis. BD is not simple chronic inflammatory disease but rather patients with BD suffer from recurrent attacks of acute inflammation in the BD lesions, where neutrophilic and lymphocytic infiltrations emerge. The etiology of BD is largely unknown, and skewed T cell responses are associated with development and maintenance of BD [1]. Excessive cytokine production by Th1 cells was reported using immunohistochemistry [2, 3] and intracellular cytokine staining [4–6]. Th1 dominance was observed in

N. Suzuki (✉) • J. Shimizu
Department of Immunology and Medicine, St. Marianna University School of Medicine, Sugao 2-16-1, Miyamae-ku, Kawasaki 216-8511, Japan
e-mail: n3suzuki@marianna-u.ac.jp

Y. Ishigatsubo (ed.), *Behçet's Disease*,
DOI 10.1007/978-4-431-54487-6_2

BD uveitis [7] and stomatitis [8]. We reported excessive Th1 cell infiltration in skin and intestinal lesions in patients with BD [9–11].

Immune responses against microbes and microbial antigens play an important role in the pathogenesis of BD. Regional differences of the disease distribution [12] suggested association of disease development with locally prevalent microbes. Oral health was often impaired in patients with BD and was correlated well with BD disease severity [13]. *Streptococcus sanguinis* is a commensal oral bacterium and often forms dental plaque. *S. sanguinis* was found frequently in oral flora in patients with BD, and the strain showed uncommon serotype (KTH1) compared with the standard ATCC strains [14]. T cells and peripheral blood mononuclear cells (PBMC) from patients with BD responded to KTH1 antigens extensively and produced interferon gamma (IFNgamma) and IL12 [15].

Recently, Th1/Th2 paradigm was challenged by the discovery of various subsets of Th cells, such as Th17 cells and regulatory T (Treg) cells [16] (Fig. 2.1). Researchers showed that Th cell differentiation in each subset was closely related and sometimes converted into the other subset in response to environmental signals both in peripheral blood and in organs [17]. Recent studies on innate immune system suggested that antigen-presenting cells (APC) stimulated with pattern recognition receptors (PRR) and corresponding ligands, including microbe antigens, regulated Th cell differentiation by cytokine production [18]. We summarize current understanding of innate and adaptive immune functions in patients with BD, especially in view of IL12/IL23 cytokines produced by activated APC through PRR.

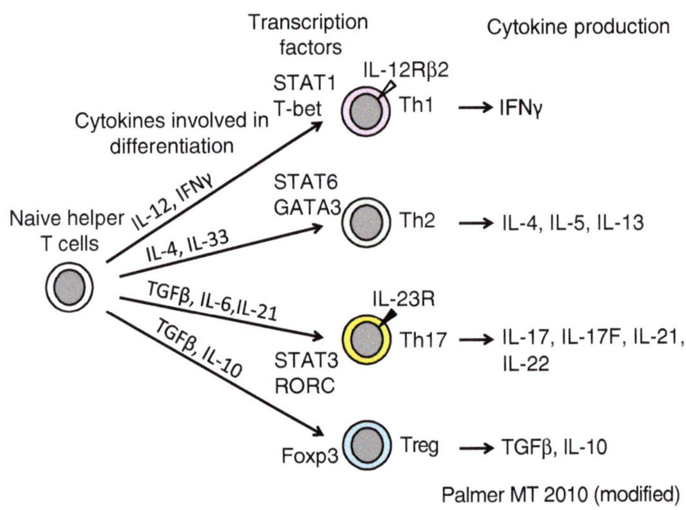

Fig. 2.1 Current view of helper T (Th) cell subsets in humans [16]
Naive Th cells differentiate into several Th cell subsets in the presence of appropriate cytokines. In response to the cytokines, the corresponding signaling molecules and transcription factors are expressed to regulate lineage commitments. Th1 and Th17 cells require IL12 and IL23 for their expansion, respectively. Foxp3: forkhead box P3, GATA: GATA transcription factor, RORC: retinoic acid receptor-related orphan receptor c, STAT: signal transducer and activator of transcription3, TGFbeta: transforming growth factor beta

2.2 Th1 Cells, Th17 Cells, Treg Cells, and IL12/IL23 Family Cytokines

2.2.1 IL12/IL23 Family Cytokines

Th17 cells produce a number of proinflammatory cytokines, including IL17, IL17F, IL21, and IL22. IL6, IL21, and transforming growth factor (TGF) beta played a role in the differentiation of Th17 cells which proliferated in the presence of IL23 (Fig. 2.1) [16]. Treg cells control T cell immune responses and also need TGFbeta for their differentiation (Fig. 2.1) [16]. TGFbeta activates Smad pathway, and activated Smad protein leads to forkhead box P3 (Foxp3) expression which is a master gene of Treg cells [19]. In the presence of TGFbeta, IL6/signal transducer and activator of transcription 3 (STAT3) signaling pathway plays a critical role in the induction of retinoic acid receptor-related orphan receptor c (RORC) expression which is a master gene of Th17 cells [20]. The two Th cell subsets require a common stimulation of TGFbeta for the cell differentiation, but the resultant cells show opposite immune function in the presence and the absence of IL6.

As mentioned above, Th17 cells require IL23 for the proliferation and survival, while Th1 cells require IL12 for the differentiation (Fig. 2.1). IL12, IL23, IL27, and IL35 are heterodimeric proteins and share their subunits partly (Fig. 2.2) [21]. IL23 is composed of p19 and p40 subunits. IL12 is composed of p35 and p40 subunits. IL35 is composed of p35 and Epstein-Barr virus-induced gene 3 (Ebi3) subunits. IL27 is composed of p28 and Ebi3 subunits. The f cytokines require each relevant receptor, some of which share their components for transducing intracellular activation signals (Fig. 2.2). IL23 receptor (IL23R) and IL12 receptor (IL12R) share IL12Ralpha subunit (IL12Ralpha), and IL12R and IL35R share IL12Rbeta subunit (IL12Rbeta). It is assumed that the 4 cytokines have partly overlapping but distinct effects on T cells with relevant Janus kinase (JAK)-STAT signaling pathway. A functional spectrum of the 4 cytokines was suggested from proinflammatory IL12 to inhibitory IL27 in Th cell differentiation (Fig. 2.2). IL23 and IL12 are produced by activated dendritic cells and macrophages and induce inflammation through Th17 and Th1 differentiation, respectively. IL23 phosphorylates STAT1, STAT3, STAT4, and STAT5. However, STAT4 activation by IL23, which is essential to produce IFNgamma, is not as strong as that by IL12 [22]. IL35 is mainly produced by Treg cells, amplifies IL35-producing Th cells, and induces T cell arrest through STAT1 and STAT4 heterodimer formation in mice [23], but the function in humans is still controversial [24]. Our preliminary experiments indicated that IL35 stimulated Th cells in a similar manner to IL12 stimulation and thus is possibly proinflammatory. IL27 is secreted from APC and produces IL10 secreting Th cells, which are suggested to inhibit local inflammation, through STAT1 and STAT3 phosphorylation [25].

Moreover, IL6 and IL11, both of which are single molecule cytokines, need gp130 for their intracellular signal transduction in Th cell differentiation [26]. The concept of IL12/IL23 family cytokine spectrum needs to be confirmed. The molecular

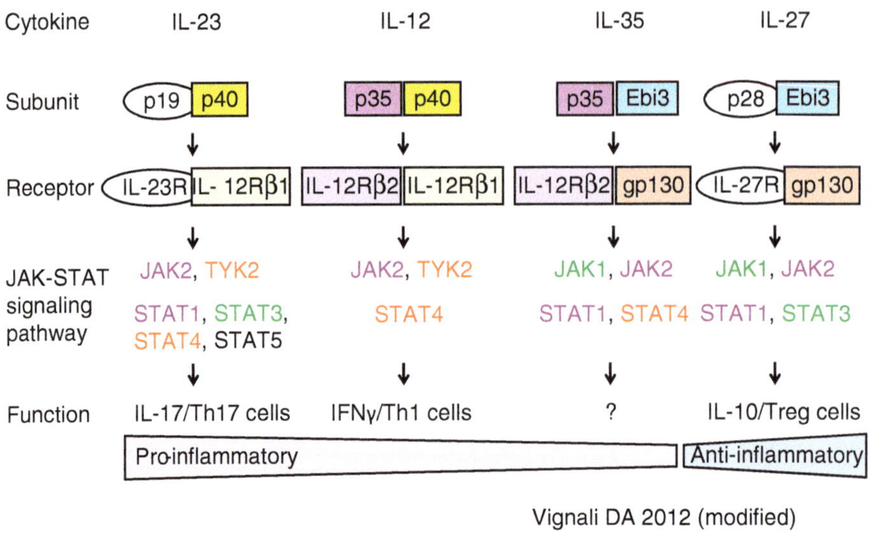

Fig. 2.2 A schematic representation of IL12/IL23 family cytokines and the corresponding receptors and JAK-STAT signaling pathways [21]
IL12, IL23, IL27, and IL35 are heterodimeric proteins and share their subunits partly. The four cytokines require each relevant receptor, some of which share their components for transducing intracellular activation signals. The four cytokines have partly overlapping but distinct effects on T cells with relevant Janus kinase (JAK)-STAT signaling pathway. A functional spectrum of the four cytokines was reported from proinflammatory IL12 to inhibitory IL27 in Th cell differentiation. IL23 and IL12 are produced by activated dendritic cells and macrophages and induce inflammation through Th17 and Th1 differentiation, respectively. IL23 phosphorylates STAT1, STAT 3, STAT 4, and STAT 5. However, STAT4 activation by IL23, which is essential to produce IFNgamma, is not as strong as that by IL12. IL35 is mainly produced by Treg cells and amplifies IL35-producing Th cells. The function of IL35 in humans is still controversial. Our preliminary experiments in humans indicated that IL35 stimulated Th cells in a similar manner to IL12 stimulation, thus is possibly proinflammatory. IL27 is secreted from APC and produces IL10-secreting Th cells, which are suggested to inhibit local inflammation, through STAT1 and STAT3 phosphorylation

mechanisms governing the IL12/IL23 family cytokine spectrum remains largely unclear. Nonetheless, it is now clear that IL12 and IL23 signaling pathways play important roles in the immune aberration in patients with BD (see below).

2.2.2 *Th1 and Th17 Cells in BD*

Th1 cytokine [2–11] and chemokine [3, 5, 10] expressions increased in peripheral blood and in lesions in patients with BD. We found that circulating and skin infiltrating lymphocytes expressed higher levels of IFNgamma and Txk protein, which regulates IFNgamma secretion, in patients with BD compared with those in normal controls and in patients with atopic dermatitis [11].

It is generally assumed that Th17 effector function increases in patients with BD. Overexpression of RORC mRNA [27, 28] and high frequencies of Th17 cells [27–29] were reported in patients with BD. Th17 cells were found in skin lesions [27, 28] and brain inflammatory lesions [29]. We recently reported that TGFbeta/ Smad signaling pathway was overactivated in peripheral circulation of patients with BD [30]. It is likely that Th cells in patients with BD show higher sensitivity to IL23 and IL12, and produce more IFNgamma and IL17, as compared with normal controls [28].

The concept that Th17 cell phenotype was solidly fixed in vitro and in vivo was turned to be not correct. Th17 cells turned into IFNgamma-expressing Th17 cells and subsequently further differentiated into nonstandard Th1 cells (Fig. 2.3) [31, 32]. The IFNgamma-expressing Th17 cells and nonstandard Th1 cells have higher affinity for inflammatory lesions than original Th17 cells and are assigned a pathophysiological role [33]. We observed Th1, Th17, and IFNgamma-expressing Th17 cells simultaneously in PBMC [28] and skin specimen obtained from erythema nodosum-like lesion [34] of BD. We speculate that Th17 cells and Th1 cells and their transition (IFNgamma-expressing Th17 cells) may associate with the pathogenesis of BD. In accordance with the hypothesis, genome-wide association studies (GWAS) suggested the importance of IL17 [35], IL23RIL12RB2 [35, 36], STAT4 [35, 37], and GTPase of the immunity-associated protein (GIMAP) [38], a Th1 cell differentiation associating GTPase, and genes for the susceptibility gene of BD.

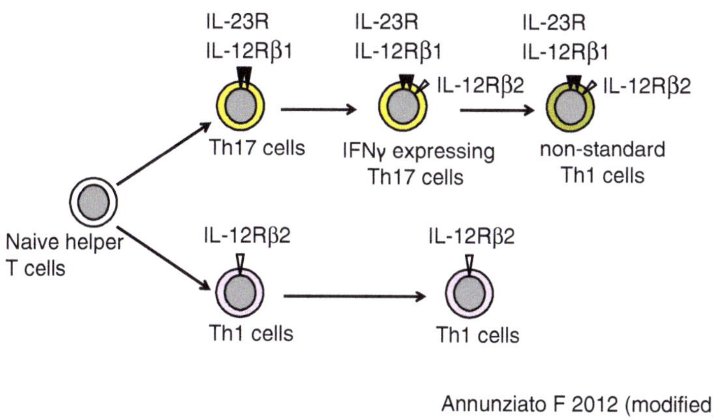

Fig. 2.3 Th17 and Th1 cell differentiations and the phenotype plasticity [31, 32]
Th17 cells turned into IFNgamma-expressing Th17 cells and subsequently further differentiated into nonstandard Th1 cells. The IFNgamma-expressing Th17 cells and nonstandard Th1 cells have higher affinity for inflammatory lesions than original Th17 cells and are assigned a pathophysiological role. IFNgamma-expressing Th17 cells were found in several human autoimmune diseases [33]. We observed Th1, Th17, and IFNgamma-expressing Th17 cells simultaneously in PBMC [28] and skin specimen obtained from erythema nodosum-like lesion [34] of BD

2.2.3 *Treg Cells in BD*

The role of Treg cells in the pathogenesis of BD is still controversial. Foxp3+ Treg cell frequencies were nearly equivalent or lower in patients with BD than those in normal controls [29, 39]. Treg cells required CD25, IL2 receptor alpha, for their survival [40], and low [41] and high [39] frequencies of CD25+ Treg cells were observed in BD patients compared with normal controls. Foxp3 gene expressions in cerebrospinal fluid [42] and CD25+ Treg cells [43] were high in BD patients compared with normal controls. It was reported that Treg cells had plasticity in the cell fate similar to Th17 cells [40], and epigenomic changes of Foxp3 gene regulated the stability [44]. The plasticity of Treg cells by the unstable expressions of Foxp3 in Th cells in patients with BD is associated with their immune aberration needs to be tested further.

2.3 B Cells and Autoantibodies in BD

2.3.1 *B Cells*

Even though hypergammaglobulinemia in patients with BD is not as prominent as that in patients with Sjögren syndrome and other collagen diseases, we reported abnormal B lymphocyte function in patients with BD almost three decades ago. In the peripheral blood, the B lymphocytes that spontaneously secrete immunoglobulins increased, yet mitogen-induced proliferation decreased [45]. Several lines of evidences support the notion. Indeed, abnormalities of B lymphocyte-driven humoral immunity have been reported. IgM and C3 have been shown to be deposited in oral ulcers and erythema nodosum-like lesions in BD patients [46]. Increases in serum immunoglobulin and autoantibodies, such as antinuclear antibodies and anti-endothelial cell antibodies, have been reported [47]. Plasma cells infiltrate the synovial tissue in BD, and apparent germinal centers are observed in the arthritic tissue [48, 49]. Frequencies of peripheral activated (CD80+) and memory (CD45RO+) B cells increased in patients with BD [50]. Immunoglobulin overproduction was observed in an assay of Epstein-Barr virus-induced B cell activation with autologous T cell stimulation [51]. Serum [52] and bronchoalveolar fluid [53] levels of B cell-activating factor of the TNF family (BAFF) were elevated in patients with BD. The bronchoalveolar fluid BAFF levels had a significant relationship with IL13 concentrations of the fluid in the patients [54]. B cell infiltration into vascular wall was found in central nervous system [54] and ruptured pulmonary artery [55] in patients with BD. These findings suggest that B lymphocytes are involved in the pathophysiology of BD.

2.3.2 *Autoantibodies*

High positive rate of antibody to anti-alpha-enolase, a target antigen of anti-endothelial cell antibody (AECA), was observed in patients with BD [56]. Kinectin [57], a microtubule associated protein, and cofilin1 [58], a family of actin-binding proteins, were identified as autoantigens in patients with BD. Higher titers of anti-tropomyosin antibody were found in BD patients with posterior uveitis compared with normal controls and patients with other types of uveitis [59]. These findings support the notion that autoantibodies play a role in the development of BD symptoms and thus pathophysiology of BD.

2.4 PRR and Pathogen-/Damage-Associated Molecular Patterns (PAMP/DAMP)

2.4.1 *APC Activation Though PRR and PAMP/DAMP*

Phagocytes were activated by various pathogens and pathogen-derived antigens in innate immune responses. Recent studies provided evidence for the existence of specific receptors on the phagocytes against the microbial antigens, and they are named PRR. Structures of the receptors retain germ-line configuration and do not have a step of rearrangement throughout the cell fate even when the receptors are utilized in adaptive immune system. They recognize bacterial and viral pieces, known as pathogen-associated molecular patterns (PAMP). PAMP are indispensable parts of the microbes, such as bacterial DNA/heat-shock proteins (HSP) and viral DNA/RNA [60]. Interaction between PRR and PAMP and subsequent induction of innate immune functions are highly conserved among various species [61].

Toll-like receptors (TLR) are transmembrane glycoproteins and called membrane-associated PRR. 10 functional human TLR have been identified [62]. TLR recognize major PAMP and also react with endogenous damage-associated molecular patterns (DAMP) secreted from severe damaged host cells caused by environmental stress, such as microbial infection and injury. DAMP include self-DNA/self-RNA and self-HSP [63]. Major TLR, PAMP, and DAMP were summarized in Table 2.1.

Two major TLR signaling pathways were demonstrated, namely, myeloid differentiation primary response protein (MyD)88-dependent pathway and Toll/interleukin receptor 1 (TIR) domain-containing adaptor-inducing IFNbeta (TRIF)-dependent pathway (Fig. 2.4). With TLR stimulation, except TLR3, APC produced proinflammatory cytokines through MyD88 and activated mitogen-activated protein kinases (MAPK, Fig. 2.4a). APC produced type 1 IFN by utilizing TRIF through TLR3 stimulation, an intracellular TLR (Fig. 2.4b) [61].

Table 2.1 Pattern recognition receptor (PRR) and corresponding PAMP and DAMP [65, 67]

TLR	PAMP	DAMP
TLR1	Bacterial lipopeptide	
TLR2	HSP (mycobacteria, chlamydia), LPS, bacterial lipopeptide, peptidoglycan	HSP, HMGB1, lipoprotein
TLR3	Viral RNA	Self-RNA
TLR4	HSP (mycobacteria, chlamydia), LPS	HSP60, HSP70, lipoprotein
TLR6	Bacterial lipopeptide	
TLR7	Viral and bacterial RNA	Chromatin and ribonucleoprotein, self-DNA
TLR9	Viral, bacterial, and parasitic DNA	HSP, chromatin and ribonucleoprotein, self-DNA
NOD	Bacterial peptidoglycan fragments	
NALP3	Bacterial RNA and ATP	Uric acid crystals, cholesterol crystals, ROS

ATP adenosine triphosphate, *DAMP* damage-associated molecular patterns, *HSP* heat-shock proteins, *LPS* lipopolysaccharide, *NALP* NACHT, LRR, and PYD domains-containing protein, *NOD* nucleotide-binding oligomerization domain-containing protein, *PAMP* pathogen-associated molecular patterns, *PRR* pattern recognition receptors, *ROS* reactive oxygen species, *TLR* Toll-like receptors

Structures of PRR retain germ-line configuration and do not have a step of rearrangement throughout the cell fate and recognize bacterial and viral pieces, known as PAMP. PAMP are indispensable parts of the microbes, such as LPS, peptidoglycan, bacterial DNA/HSP, and viral DNA/RNA. Interaction between PRR and PAMP and subsequent induction of innate immune function are highly conserved among species

PRR also recognize endogenous DAMP which are secreted from severe damaged host cells caused by any environmental stress, such as microbial infection or injury. DAMP include self-DNA/self-RNA and self-HSP. These molecules were reported to be rapidly released following unprogrammed cell death and activate PRR-expressing cells similar to the PAMP

In PAMP, bacterial lipopeptides, HSP, and LPS were recognized by TLR1/TLR2/TLR6, TLR2/TLR4, and TLR4 with CD14, respectively. Similar mechanisms were found in DAMP with self-lipoproteins and self-HSP

Nucleotide-binding oligomerization domain (NOD)-like receptors are major intracellular PRR. NOD proteins recognize bacterial peptidoglycan fragments, and NALP3 is involved in the recognition of bacterial RNA/ATP

2.4.2 T Cell Differentiation Through PRR Stimulation

2.4.2.1 HSP as a Major TLR Ligand of Th Cells

Upon stimulation with TLR4, dendritic cells produced p19, p35, p40, p28, and Ebi3 [64–68], all of which are IL12/IL23 family cytokine subunits and mediate pro- and anti-inflammatory effects (Fig. 2.2), for several hours in succession. The TLR4-stimulated dendritic cells may regulate positively and negatively T cell differentiation toward Th1/Th17 cells and IL10/Treg cells by secretion of IL12/IL23 family cytokines [21, 25].

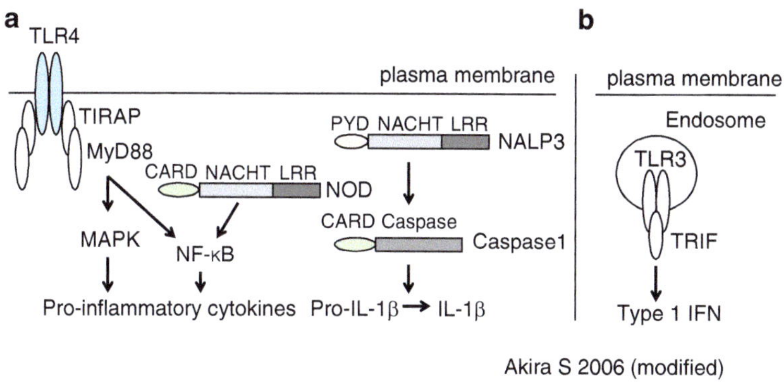

Fig. 2.4 Major TLR and NOD-like receptor signaling pathways [61]
TLR4 was expressed on phagocyte cell surfaces and TLR3 localized within intracellular vesicles. Cell surface TLR recognized cell membrane-type PAMP. Intracellular TLR recognized nucleic acid-type PAMP. (**a**) With TLR stimulation, except TLR3, APC produced proinflammatory cytokines through MyD88 and activated MAPK. NOD-like receptors are major intracellular PRR. NOD proteins recognize bacterial peptidoglycan fragments and activate NF-kappaB to produce proinflammatory cytokines. NACHT, LRR, and PYD domains-containing protein 3 (NALP3) is involved in the recognition of bacterial RNA/adenosine triphosphate and is a major component of NALP3 inflammasome, the activation of which promotes digestion of proIL1beta into functionally mature truncated IL1beta with activated Caspase1. (**b**) APC produced type 1 IFN by utilizing of TRIF through TLR3 stimulation, an intracellular TLR
CARD: Caspase recruitment domain, IFN: interferon, LRR: leucine-rich repeat, MAPK: mitogen-activated protein kinases, MyD88: myeloid differentiation primary response protein 88, NACHT: neuronal apoptosis inhibitory protein (NAIP), Class II, major histocompatibility complex, transactivator (CIITA), HET-E, TP1, NF-kappaB: nuclear factor kappa-light-chain-enhancer of activated B cells, NOD: nucleotide-binding oligomerization domain, PYD: pyrin domain, TIRAP: Toll/interleukin 1 receptor (TIR) domain-containing adaptor protein, TRIF: TIR domain-containing adaptor-inducing IFNbeta

Intracellular signaling pathway of Th cells activated by TLR2 and TLR4 stimulation converges with T cell receptor (TCR) signaling pathway [18]. TCR stimulation activates T cells by phosphorylation of extracellular signal-regulated kinases (ERK) 1 and 2 which are subsets of MAPK family. TLR stimulation regulated Th cell activation mainly by the interference of the ERK phosphorylation (Fig. 2.5) [18, 67].

HSP are highly conserved and ubiquitously expressed proteins and function as an intracellular chaperonin for other proteins. The first study reported that "heat shock" remarkably increased an HSP expression in Drosophila salivary glands [68]. Numerous studies named subgroups of HSP for their molecular weights and subdivided their functions into two major systems. HSP60-HSP10 system assisted the adequate protein folding and HSP70-HSP40 system was involved in the stability of cytosolic peptides [69]. Significant sequence homology is found between mammalian and microbial HSP. For example, mycobacterial and streptococcal HSP65 have more than 90 % homology, and mycobacterial HSP65 and human HSP60 have 42 % homology [70].

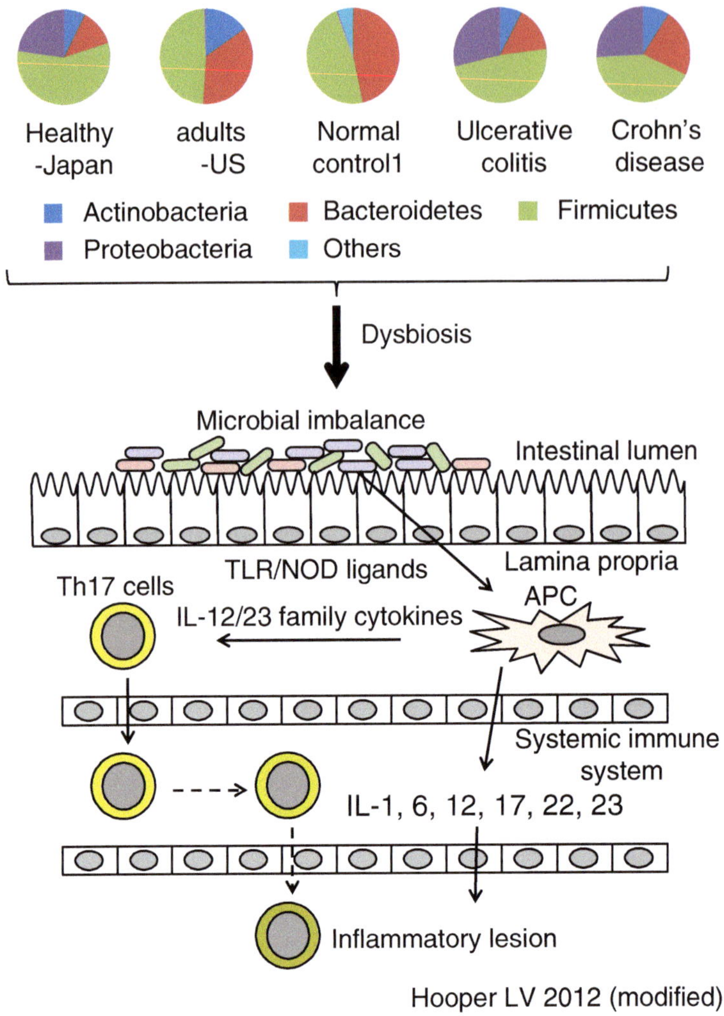

Fig. 2.5 A hypothesis of immunopathogenesis in patients with BD: imbalance of microorganisms regulates aberrant Th cell differentiation, leading to the development of the disease
New assessment of gut microbes with genome DNA sequence technique is used to investigate the relationship between gut microbiota and human immune diseases. It was reported that *Clostridium* family in phylum *Firmicutes* was reduced and *Bacteroidetes* and *Proteobacteria* species increase in patients with inflammatory bowel diseases [104–107]
The intestinal microbial imbalance, so called dysbiosis, has been shown to induce systemic and local immune response through both innate and adaptive immune cells. Massive accumulation of APC with IL12/IL23 family cytokines in lamina propria and corresponding (possibly pathogenic) microbes in the lumen may provoke systemic activation of APC and subsequently high frequency of Th17 cells in systemic immune system. This type of immune aberration may cause adjacent inflammation (GI tract) and remote lesions, such as uveitis, in patients with BD with undisclosed mechanisms. We need to clarify the relationship between the frequency and diversity of GI tract microbes and Th cell function in patients with BD

Microbes and necrotic cells secreted HSP and APC recognized them through TLR2 and TLR4 [61]. HSP were categorized into both PAMP and DAMP (Table 2.1) [63, 71]. Certainly, clinical studies demonstrated that HSP accumulation promoted and exaggerated the lesions of several human autoimmune diseases [72]. On the contrary, several experimental model studies of autoimmunity reported protective effects of HSP peptide by deletion of peptide-specific T cells [73]. Oral administration of an HSP peptide reduced disease activity in patients with rheumatoid arthritis [74].

2.4.2.2 HSP Expression in BD

Both TLR and HSP expressions increased in patients with BD. Elevated gene expressions of TLR2 and TLR4 were found in peripheral blood monocytes [75], PBMC [76], polymorphonuclear leukocytes [76], bronchoalveolar lavage leukocytes [77], and oral mucosa [78] in patients with BD. TLR2- and TLR4-positive cells in buccal lesions [79] and TLR6-positive polymorphonuclear leukocytes after culture with HSP60 [80] significantly increased in patients with BD. Several researchers observed massive expressions of HSP60 in BD skin [81] and oral ulcer lesions [82, 83]. HSP60 was expressed more diffusely [83] and intensely [81, 83] in BD lesions than those in other types of inflammation, such as oral lichen planus and recurrent aphthous stomatitis. It is clear that HSP is expressed extensively in the lesions; thus HSP is a possible triggering antigen of immune aberration in patients with BD.

2.4.2.3 Th Cells and HSP in BD

Excessive T and B cell responses to major four peptides of Mycobacterium tuberculosis HSP65 and human counterparts of HSP60 were observed in patients with BD who lived in Europe, Middle East, and Japan along with Silk Route [11, 84, 85].

We have found that TLR2 and TLR4 mRNA were expressed on ileocecal ulcer lesions of BD but less on unaffected sites of BD and on Crohn's disease lesions. IL12 producing TLR2-positive macrophages located neighboring to T cells and HSP60 was expressed on the same region of the intestinal lesions [9, 10]. C-C type chemokine receptor (CCR)5 and macrophage inflammatory protein (MIP)1beta, a Th1-related chemokine receptor and its ligand, were detected in the intestinal lesions of BD, and CCR5/MIP1beta interaction was thought to play a role in the migration of activated Th1 cells [10]. Moreover, Th cells yielded proliferative responses to human HSP60 peptide in Japanese BD patients by antigen-driven process [85]. We suggest that TLR/HSP60 interactions induce destructive Th1 type responses at the intestinal lesion in patients with BD [86]. In accordance with the hypothesis, a targeted resequence and a GWAS identified TLR4 [87] and endoplasmic reticulum aminopeptidase 1 (ERAP1) [88], an antigen presentation associating aminopeptidase, as BD susceptibility genes, respectively.

2.4.2.4 Gammadelta T Cells and HSP in BD

Gammadelta T cells are small population of T cells and bear an innate characteristics. It was thought that Vgamma9delta2+ T cells, a major subset of gammadelta T cells of peripheral blood lymphocytes, recognized the antigens produced by bacteria [89]. Vdelta1+ gammadelta T cells responded to the stress-inducible major histocompatibility complex class I related chain A (MICA) mainly expressed on damaged intestinal epithelial cells [90]. Many types of gammadelta T cells express TLR2. Gammadelta T cells produced IL17 in the presence of TLR2 ligands and IL23, and the production was significantly reduced when the cells deprived of IL23 stimulation. It was suggested that gammadelta T cells shared some common features with Th17 cells [91].

Vdelta2+ gammadelta T cells increased in peripheral blood, while Vdelta1+ gammadelta T cells increased in bronchoalveolar lavage fluid and cerebrospinal fluid in patients with BD [92]. Gammadelta T cells obtained from BD PBMC responded significantly better to HSP peptides than those from normal controls and patients with systemic lupus erythematosus or inflammatory bowel diseases [93]. Infiltrating cells expressed HSP and gammadelta T cell numbers increased in oral ulcer in patients with BD [81, 83].

We found that CD45RA+Vgamma9delta2+ gammadelta T cells increased in BD peripheral blood lymphocytes irrespective of disease activity. The CD45RA+gammadelta T cells produced tumor necrosis factor (TNF) alpha and contained perforin granules [94]. We found that Vgamma9delta1+ gammadelta T cells preferentially responded to *S. sanguinis* derived KTH1 antigen without HLA restriction [95]. It is possible that gammadelta T cells respond to HSP and other PAMP both in peripheral blood and in affected lesions and enhance systemic and local inflammation in patients with BD.

2.5 NOD-Like Receptor Involvement in BD

Nucleotide-binding oligomerization domain (NOD)-like receptors are major intracellular PRR. NOD proteins activate nuclear factor kappa-light-chain-enhancer of activated B cells (NF-kappaB) to produce proinflammatory cytokines (Fig. 2.4a, Table 2.1) [61]. Neuronal apoptosis inhibitory protein (NAIP), Class II, major histocompatibility complex, transactivator (CIITA), HET-E, TP1 (NACHT), leucine-rich repeat (LRR) and pyrin domain (PYD) domains-containing protein 3 (NALP3) is a major component of NALP3 inflammasome, the activation of which promotes digestion of proIL1beta into functional mature truncated IL1beta with activated Caspase1 (Fig. 2.4a, Table 2.1) [61]. It was suggested that NOD-like receptors acted in synergy with TLR ligands in APC. Costimulation of NOD-like receptors and TLR7/8 promoted APC secretion of IL23 and enhanced the activation of

Th17 cells [96]. Genetically inactivated NOD2 signals ameliorated experimental arthritis with reduced levels of IL6, IL17, and IL23 in the joints [97].

Recent studies of NOD-like receptors provided new insights into the molecular mechanisms of BD pathogenesis. NOD2 but not NOD1 gene expression was significantly increased in bronchoalveolar lavage of BD patients compared with that of normal controls [77]. In contrast, APC obtained from BD patients produced lower levels of IL18, another major downstream cytokine of inflammasome signaling, than those from normal controls [98]. Moreover, IL1beta production of PBMC was significantly lower in patient with BD compared with normal controls in the presence of adenosine triphosphate and monosodium urate crystals, both of which are NALP3 ligands (Table 2.1) [99]. Serum IL1beta levels were significantly higher in patients with BD than those in normal controls [100, 101], and several antibodies against IL1beta were effective in treating BD patients with refractory uveitis [102, 103]. Further investigations are needed to elucidate the role of NOD-like receptor in the pathogenesis of BD.

2.6 Conclusions and Perspective

Skewed Th1/Th17 responses and production of IL12/IL23 cytokines may be important in the pathophysiological conditions in BD. TCR and PRR signaling pathways may have distinct effects on the development of Th1, Th17, Treg, and gammadelta T cells.

The relationship between the distribution of IL12/IL23 cytokines and each Th cell subsets needs to be studied. Mucosal immune response was thought to be a candidate for providing both effector and regulatory immunological function to the lesion. Commensal bacteria regulated Th cell differentiation of both Th17 cells and Treg cells mainly through TLR/NOD ligands [104]. We suggest that massive accumulation of APC with IL12/IL23 cytokines in lamina propria and corresponding pathogenic microbes in the lumen cause systemic activation of APC, high frequency of Th17 cells in systemic immune system, and inflammation of the lesions in patients with BD (Fig. 2.5).

Recently, new assessment of gut commensal bacteria with next-generation sequence technology has been established. This technique, so called metagenomics, allows nearly complete genome assembly from individual microbes directly from clinical samples, such as fetus (Fig. 2.5) [105–107]. We now investigate the relationship between the metagenomic sequence data of gut microbes from BD patient and their T cell function to develop new therapeutic strategy in patients with BD.

Acknowledgement Our works were supported in part by grants from Behçet's Disease Research Committee, Research on Specific Disease of the Health Science Research Grants from the Ministry of Health, Labor and Welfare, Japan.

References

1. Sakane T, Takeno M, Suzuki N, Inaba G. Behçet's disease. N Engl J Med. 1999;341:1284–91.
2. Melikoglu M, Uysal S, Krueger JG, et al. Characterization of the divergent wound-healing responses occurring in the pathergy reaction and normal healthy volunteers. J Immunol. 2006;177:6415–21.
3. Ben Ahmed M, Houman H, Miled M, Dellagi K, Louzir H. Involvement of chemokines and Th1 cytokines in the pathogenesis of mucocutaneous lesions of Behçet's disease. Arthritis Rheum. 2004;50:2291–5.
4. Koarada S, Haruta Y, Tada Y, et al. Increased entry of CD4+ T cells into the Th1 cytokine effector pathway during T-cell division following stimulation in Behcet's disease. Rheumatology (Oxford). 2004;43:843–51.
5. Houman H, Hamzaoui A, Ben Ghorbal I, Khanfir M, Feki M, Hamzaoui K. Abnormal expression of chemokine receptors in Behçet's disease: relationship to intracellular Th1/Th2 cytokines and to clinical manifestations. J Autoimmun. 2004;23:267–73.
6. Frassanito MA, Dammacco R, Cafforio P, Dammacco F. Th1 polarization of the immune response in Behçet's disease: a putative pathogenetic role of interleukin-12. Arthritis Rheum. 1999;42:1967–74.
7. Ilhan F, Demir T, Türkçüoğlu P, Turgut B, Demir N, Gödekmerdan A. Th1 polarization of the immune response in uveitis in Behçet's disease. Can J Ophthalmol. 2008;43:105–8.
8. Dalghous AM, Freysdottir J, Fortune F. Expression of cytokines, chemokines, and chemokine receptors in oral ulcers of patients with Behcet's disease (BD) and recurrent aphthous stomatitis is Th1-associated, although Th2-association is also observed in patients with BD. Scand J Rheumatol. 2006;35:472–5.
9. Nara K, Kurokawa MS, Chiba S, et al. Involvement of innate immunity in the pathogenesis of intestinal Behçet's disease. Clin Exp Immunol. 2008;152:245–51.
10. Imamura Y, Kurokawa MS, Yoshikawa H, et al. Involvement of Th1 cells and heat shock protein 60 in the pathogenesis of intestinal Behcet's disease. Clin Exp Immunol. 2005;139:371–8.
11. Nagafuchi H, Takeno M, Yoshikawa H, et al. Excessive expression of Txk, a member of the Tec family of tyrosine kinases, contributes to excessive Th1 cytokine production by T lymphocytes in patients with Behcet's disease. Clin Exp Immunol. 2005;139:363–70.
12. Choe JY, Chung WT, Lee SW, et al. Regional distinction for the clinical severity of Behçet's disease in Korea: four university-based medical centers study. Clin Exp Rheumatol. 2010;28:S20–26.
13. Mumcu G, Ergun T, Inanc N, et al. Oral health is impaired in Behçet's disease and is associated with disease severity. Rheumatology (Oxford). 2004;43:1028–33.
14. Yokota K, Hayashi S, Araki Y, et al. Characterization of Streptococcus sanguis isolated from patients with Behçet's disease. Microbiol Immunol. 1995;39:729–32.
15. Yanagihori H, Oyama N, Nakamura K, Mizuki N, Oguma K, Kaneko F. Role of IL12B promoter polymorphism in Adamantiades-Behcet's disease susceptibility: an involvement of Th1 immunoreactivity against *Streptococcus sanguinis* antigen. J Invest Dermatol. 2006;126:1534–40.
16. Palmer MT, Weaver CT. Autoimmunity: increasing suspects in the CD4+ T cell lineup. Nat Immunol. 2010;11:36–40.
17. Basu R, Hatton RD, Weaver CT. The Th17 family: flexibility follows function. Immunol Rev. 2013;252:89–103.
18. Reynolds JM, Dong C. Toll-like receptor regulation of effector T lymphocyte function. Trends Immunol. 2013;34:511–9.
19. Lu L, Wang J, Zhang F, et al. Role of SMAD and non-SMAD signals in the development of Th17 and regulatory T cells. J Immunol. 2010;184:4295–306.

20. Bettelli E, Carrier Y, Gao W, et al. Reciprocal developmental pathways for the generation of pathogenic effector TH17 and regulatory T cells. Nature. 2006;441:235–8.
21. Vignali DA, Kuchroo VK. IL12 family cytokines: immunological playmakers. Nat Immunol. 2012;13:722–8.
22. Parham C, Chirica M, Timans J, et al. A receptor for the heterodimeric cytokine IL23 is composed of IL12Rbeta1 and a novel cytokine receptor subunit, IL23R. J Immunol. 2002;168:5699–708.
23. Stumhofer JS, Silver JS, Laurence A, et al. Interleukins 27 and 6 induce STAT3-mediated T cell production of interleukin 10. Nat Immunol. 2007;8:1363–71.
24. Collison LW, Workman CJ, Kuo TT, et al. The inhibitory cytokine IL35 contributes to regulatory T-cell function. Nature. 2007;450:566–9.
25. Bardel E, Larousserie F, Charlot-Rabiega P, Coulomb-L'Herminé A, Devergne O. Human CD4+ CD25+ Foxp3+ regulatory T cells do not constitutively express IL35. J Immunol. 2008;181:6898–905.
26. Garbers C, Hermanns HM, Schaper F, et al. Plasticity and cross-talk of interleukin 6-type cytokines. Cytokine Growth Factor Rev. 2012;23:85–97.
27. Hamzaoui K, Bouali E, Ghorbel I, Khanfir M, Houman H, Hamzaoui A. Expression of Th-17 and RORγt mRNA in Behçet's Disease. Med Sci Monit. 2011;17:CR227–234.
28. Shimizu J, Takai K, Fujiwara N, et al. Excessive CD4+ T cells co-expressing interleukin-17 and interferon-γ in patients with Behçet's disease. Clin Exp Immunol. 2012;168:68–74.
29. Geri G, Terrier B, Rosenzwajg M, et al. Critical role of IL21 in modulating TH17 and regulatory T cells in Behçet disease. J Allergy Clin Immunol. 2011;128:655–64.
30. Shimizu J, Izumi T, Arimitsu N, et al. Skewed TGFβ/Smad signalling pathway in T cells in patients with Behçet's disease. Clin Exp Rheumatol. 2012;30:S35–39.
31. Muranski P, Restifo NP. Essentials of Th17 cell commitment and plasticity. Blood. 2013;121:2402–14.
32. Annunziato F, Cosmi L, Liotta F, Maggi E, Romagnani S. Defining the human T helper 17 cell phenotype. Trends Immunol. 2012;33:505–12.
33. Annunziato F, Cosmi L, Santarlasci V, et al. Phenotypic and functional features of human Th17 cells. J Exp Med. 2007;204:1849–61.
34. Shimizu J, Kaneko F, Suzuki N. Skewed helper T cell responses to IL12 family cytokines produced by antigen presenting cells and the genetic background in Behcet's disease. Genet Res Int. 2013. doi:10.1155/2013/363859.
35. Kim ES, Kim SW, Moon CM, et al. Interactions between IL17A, IL23R, and STAT4 polymorphisms confer susceptibility to intestinal Behcet's disease in Korean population. Life Sci. 2012;90:740–6.
36. Xavier JM, Shahram F, Davatchi F, et al. Association study of IL10 and IL23RIL12RB2 in Iranian patients with Behçet's disease. Arthritis Rheum. 2012;64:2761–72.
37. Hou S, Yang Z, Du L, et al. Identification of a susceptibility locus in STAT4 for Behçet's disease in Han Chinese in a genome-wide association study. Arthritis Rheum. 2012;64:4104–13.
38. Lee YJ, Horie Y, Wallace GR, et al. Genome-wide association study identifies GIMAP as a novel susceptibility locus for Behcet's disease. Ann Rheum Dis. 2013;72:1510–6.
39. Pekiner FN, Aytugar E, Demirel GY, Borahan MO. Interleukin-2, interleukin-6 and T regulatory cells in peripheral blood of patients with Behçet's disease and recurrent aphthous ulcerations. J Oral Pathol Med. 2012;41:73–9.
40. Sakaguchi S, Vignali DA, Rudensky AY, Niec RE, Waldmann H. The plasticity and stability of regulatory T cells. Nat Rev Immunol. 2013;13:461–7.
41. Nanke Y, Kotake S, Goto M, Ujihara H, Matsubara M, Kamatani N. Decreased percentages of regulatory T cells in peripheral blood of patients with Behcet's disease before ocular attack: a possible predictive marker of ocular attack. Mod Rheumatol. 2008;18:354–8.
42. Hamzaoui K, Borhani Haghighi A, Ghorbel IB, Houman H. RORC and Foxp3 axis in cerebrospinal fluid of patients with neuro-Behçet's disease. J Neuroimmunol. 2011;233:249–53.

43. Hamzaoui K, Hamzaoui A, Houman H. CD4+CD25+ regulatory T cells in patients with Behçet's disease. Clin Exp Rheumatol. 2006;24:S71–78.
44. Ohkura N, Kitagawa Y, Sakaguchi S. Development and maintenance of regulatory T cells. Immunity. 2013;38:414–23.
45. Suzuki N, Sakane T, Ueda Y, Tsunematsu T. Abnormal B cell function in patients with Behçet's disease. Arthritis Rheum. 1986;29:212–9.
46. Kaneko F, Takahashi Y, Muramatsu Y, Miura Y. Immunological studies on aphthous ulcer and erythema nodosum-like eruptions in Behçet's disease. Br J Dermatol. 1985;113:303–12.
47. Taylor PV, Chamberlain MA, Scott JS. Autoreactivity in patients with Behçet's disease. Br J Rheumatol. 1993;32:908–10.
48. Yurdakul S, Yazici H, Tuzun Y, Pazarli H, Yalcin B, Altac M, et al. The arthritis of Behçet's disease: a prospective study. Ann Rheum Dis. 1983;42:505–12.
49. Gibson T, Laurent R, Highton J, Wilton M, Dyson M, Millis R. Synovial histopathology of Behçet's syndrome. Ann Rheum Dis. 1981;40:376–81.
50. Ekşioglu-Demiralp E, Kibaroglu A, Direskeneli H, et al. Phenotypic characteristics of B cells in Behçet's disease: increased activity in B cell subsets. J Rheumatol. 1999;26:826–32.
51. Hamzaoui K, Kahan A, Hamza M, Ayed K. Suppressive T cell function of Epstein-Barr virus induced B cell activation in active Behçet's disease. Clin Exp Rheumatol. 1991;9:131–5.
52. Hamzaoui K, Houman H, Ben Dhifallah I, Kamoun M, Hamzaoui A. Serum BAFF levels and skin mRNA expression in patients with Behçet's disease. Clin Exp Rheumatol. 2008;26:S64–71.
53. Hamzaoui A, Chelbi H, Sassi FH, Hamzaoui K. Release of B cell-activating factor of the TNF family in bronchoalveolar lavage from Behçet's disease with pulmonary involvement. Oxid Med Cell Longev. 2010;3:122–8.
54. Hirohata S, Kikuchi H. Histopathology of the ruptured pulmonary artery aneurysm in a patient with Behçet's disease. Clin Exp Rheumatol. 2009;27:S91–95.
55. Hirohata S. Histopathology of central nervous system lesions in Behçet's disease. J Neurol Sci. 2008;267:41–7.
56. Lee KH, Chung HS, Kim HS, et al. Human alpha-enolase from endothelial cells as a target antigen of anti-endothelial cell antibody in Behçet's disease. Arthritis Rheum. 2003;48:2025–35.
57. Lu Y, Ye P, Chen SL, Tan EM, Chan EK. Identification of kinectin as a novel Behçet's disease autoantigen. Arthritis Res Ther. 2005;7:R1133–1139.
58. Ooka S, Nakano H, Matsuda T, et al. Proteomic surveillance of autoantigens in patients with Behcet's disease by a proteomic approach. Microbiol Immunol. 2010;54:354–61.
59. Mahesh SP, Li Z, Buggage R, et al. Alpha tropomyosin as a self-antigen in patients with Behçet's disease. Clin Exp Immunol. 2005;140:368–75.
60. Osterloh A, Breloer M. Heat shock proteins: linking danger and pathogen recognition. Med Microbiol Immunol. 2008;197:1–8.
61. Akira S, Uematsu S, Takeuchi O. Pathogen recognition and innate immunity. Cell. 2006;124:783–801.
62. Kawai T, Akira S. Toll-like receptors and their crosstalk with other innate receptors in infection and immunity. Immunity. 2011;34:637–50.
63. Piccinini AM, Midwood KS. DAMPening inflammation by modulating TLR signalling. Mediat Inflamm. 2010;2010:1–21. doi:10.1155/2010/672395.
64. Johnson J, Molle C, Aksoy E, Goldman M, Goriely S, Willems F. A conventional protein kinase C inhibitor targeting IRF-3-dependent genes differentially regulates IL12 family members. Mol Immunol. 2011;48:1484–93.
65. Jackson AM, Mulcahy LA, Porte J, et al. Role of mitogen-activated protein kinase and PI3K pathways in the regulation of IL12-family cytokines in dendritic cells and the generation of T H-responses. Eur Cytokine Netw. 2010;21:319–28.

66. Schuetze N, Schoeneberger S, Mueller U, Freudenberg MA, Alber G, Straubinger RK. IL12 family members: differential kinetics of their TLR4-mediated induction by Salmonella enteritidis and the impact of IL10 in bone marrow-derived macrophages. Int Immunol. 2005;17:649–59.
67. Chapman NM, Bilal MY, Cruz-Orcutt N, et al. Distinct signaling pathways regulate TLR2 co-stimulatory function in human T cells. Cell Signal. 2013;25:639–50.
68. Ritossa F. A new puffing pattern induced by temperature shock and DNP in drosophila. Experientia. 1962;18:571–3.
69. Young JC, Agashe VR, Siegers K, Hartl FU. Pathways of chaperone-mediated protein folding in the cytosol. Nat Rev Mol Cell Biol. 2004;5:781–91.
70. Dudani AK, Gupta RS. Immunological characterization of a human homolog of the 65-kilodalton mycobacterial antigen. Infect Immun. 1989;57:2786–93.
71. Chen GY, Nuñez G. Sterile inflammation: sensing and reacting to damage. Nat Rev Immunol. 2010;10:826–37.
72. Puga Yung GL, Fidler M, Albani E, et al. Heat shock protein-derived T-cell epitopes contribute to autoimmune inflammation in pediatric Crohn's disease. PLoS One. 2009;4(11):e7714. doi:10.1371/journal.pone.0007714.
73. Zonneveld-Huijssoon E, Albani S, Prakken BJ, van Wijk F. Heat shock protein bystander antigens for peptide immunotherapy in autoimmune disease. Clin Exp Immunol. 2013;171:20–9.
74. Koffeman EC, Genovese M, Amox D, et al. Epitope-specific immunotherapy of rheumatoid arthritis: clinical responsiveness occurs with immune deviation and relies on the expression of a cluster of molecules associated with T cell tolerance in a double-blind, placebo-controlled, pilot phase II trial. Arthritis Rheum. 2009;60:3207–16.
75. Do JE, Kwon SY, Park S, Lee ES. Effects of vitamin D on expression of Toll-like receptors of monocytes from patients with Behcet's disease. Rheumatology (Oxford). 2008;47:840–8.
76. Kirino Y, Takeno M, Watanabe R, et al. Association of reduced heme oxygenase-1 with excessive Toll-like receptor 4 expression in peripheral blood mononuclear cells in Behçet's disease. Arthritis Res Ther. 2008;10(1):R16. doi:10.1186/ar2367.
77. Hamzaoui K, Abid H, Berraies A, Ammar J, Hamzaoui A. NOD2 is highly expressed in Behçet disease with pulmonary manifestations. J Inflamm (Lond). 2012;9(1):3. doi:10.1186/1476-9255-9-3.
78. Seoudi N, Bergmeier LA, Hagi-Pavli E, Bibby D, Curtis MA, Fortune F. The role of TLR2 and 4 in Behcet's disease pathogenesis. Innate Immun. 2013;20(4):412–22. doi:10.1177/1753425913498042.
79. Durrani O, Banahan K, Sheedy FJ, et al. TIRAP Ser180Leu polymorphism is associated with Behcet's disease. Rheumatology (Oxford). 2011;50:1760–5.
80. Yavuz S, Elbir Y, Tulunay A, Eksioglu-Demiralp E, Direskeneli H. Differential expression of toll-like receptor 6 on granulocytes and monocytes implicates the role of microorganisms in Behcet's disease etiopathogenesis. Rheumatol Int. 2008;28:401–6.
81. Ergun T, Ince U, Ekşioğlu-Demiralp E, et al. HSP 60 expression in mucocutaneous lesions of Behçet's disease. J Am Acad Dermatol. 2001;45:904–9.
82. Deniz E, Guc U, Buyukbabani N, Gul A. HSP 60 expression in recurrent oral ulcerations of Behçet's disease. Oral Surg Oral Med Oral Pathol Oral Radiol Endod. 2010;110:196–200.
83. Bramanti TE, Dekker NP, Lozada-Nur F, Sauk JJ, Regezi JA. Heat shock (stress) proteins and gamma delta T lymphocytes in oral lichen planus. Oral Surg Oral Med Oral Pathol Oral Radiol Endod. 1995;80:698–704.
84. Pervin K, Childerstone A, Shinnick T, et al. T cell epitope expression of mycobacterial and homologous human 65-kilodalton heat shock protein peptides in short term cell lines from patients with Behçet's disease. J Immunol. 1993;151:2273–82.
85. Kaneko S, Suzuki N, Yamashita N, et al. Characterization of T cells specific for an epitope of human 60-kD heat shock protein (hsp) in patients with Behcet's disease (BD) in Japan. Clin Exp Immunol. 1997;108:204–12.

86. Shimizu J, Izumi T, Suzuki N. Aberrant Activation of Heat Shock Protein 60/65 Reactive T Cells in Patients with Behcet's Disease. Autoimmun Dis. 2012;1(1):105205. doi:10.1155/2012/105205.
87. Kirino Y, Zhou Q, Ishigatsubo Y, et al. Targeted resequencing implicates the familial Mediterranean fever gene MEFV and the toll-like receptor 4 gene TLR4 in Behçet disease. Proc Natl Acad Sci U S A. 2013;110:8134–9.
88. Kirino Y, Bertsias G, Ishigatsubo Y, et al. Genome-wide association analysis identifies new susceptibility loci for Behçet's disease and epistasis between HLA-B*51 and ERAP1. Nat Genet. 2010;45:202–7.
89. Altincicek B, Moll J, Campos N, et al. Cutting edge: human gamma delta T cells are activated by intermediates of the 2-C-methyl-D-erythritol 4-phosphate pathway of isoprenoid biosynthesis. J Immunol. 2001;166:3655–8.
90. Groh V, Steinle A, Bauer S, Spies T. Recognition of stress-induced MHC molecules by intestinal epithelial gammadelta T cells. Science. 1998;279:1737–40.
91. Martin B, Hirota K, Cua DJ, Stockinger B, Veldhoen M. Interleukin-17-producing gammadelta T cells selectively expand in response to pathogen products and environmental signals. Immunity. 2009;31:321–30.
92. Hamzaoui K, Hamzaoui A, Hentati F, et al. Phenotype and functional profile of T cells expressing gamma delta receptor from patients with active Behçet's disease. J Rheumatol. 1994;21:2301–6.
93. Hasan A, Fortune F, Wilson A, et al. Role of gamma delta T cells in pathogenesis and diagnosis of Behcet's disease. Lancet. 1996;347:789–94.
94. Yamashita N, Kaneoka H, Kaneko S, et al. Role of gammadelta T lymphocytes in the development of Behçet's disease. Clin Exp Immunol. 1997;107:241–7.
95. Mochizuki M, Suzuki N, Takeno M, et al. Fine antigen specificity of human gamma delta T cell lines (V gamma 9+) established by repetitive stimulation with a serotype (KTH-1) of a gram-positive bacterium, Streptococcus sanguis. Eur J Immunol. 1994;24:1536–43.
96. Schwarz H, Posselt G, Wurm P, Ulbing M, Duschl A, Horejs-Hoeck J. TLR8 and NOD signaling synergistically induce the production of IL1β and IL23 in monocyte-derived DCs and enhance the expression of the feedback inhibitor SOCS2. Immunobiology. 2013;218:533–42.
97. Vieira SM, Cunha TM, França RF, et al. Joint NOD2/RIPK2 signaling regulates IL17 axis and contributes to the development of experimental arthritis. J Immunol. 2012;188:5116–22.
98. Türe-Özdemir F, Tulunay A, Elbasi MO, et al. Proinflammatory cytokine and caspase-1 responses to pattern recognition receptor activation of neutrophils and dendritic cells in Behcet's disease. Rheumatology (Oxford). 2013;52:800–5.
99. Woo MY, Cho O, Lee MJ, Kim K, Lee ES, Park S. Differential effects of colchicine in blood mononuclear cells of patients with Behçet disease in relation to colchicine responsiveness. Br J Dermatol. 2012;167:914–21.
100. Düzgün N, Ayaşlioğlu E, Tutkak H, Aydintuğ OT. Cytokine inhibitors: soluble tumor necrosis factor receptor 1 and interleukin-1 receptor antagonist in Behçet's disease. Rheumatol Int. 2005;25:1–5.
101. Yosipovitch G, Shohat B, Bshara J, Wysenbeek A, Weinberger A. Elevated serum interleukin 1 receptors and interleukin 1B in patients with Behçet's disease: correlations with disease activity and severity. Isr J Med Sci. 1995;31:345–8.
102. Gül A, Tugal-Tutkun I, Dinarello CA, et al. Interleukin-1β-regulating antibody XOMA 052 (gevokizumab) in the treatment of acute exacerbations of resistant uveitis of Behcet's disease: an open-label pilot study. Ann Rheum Dis. 2012;71:563–6.
103. Ugurlu S, Ucar D, Seyahi E, Hatemi G, Yurdakul S. Canakinumab in a patient with juvenile Behcet's syndrome with refractory eye disease. Ann Rheum Dis. 2012;71:1589–91.
104. Hooper LV, Littman DR, Macpherson AJ. Interactions between the microbiota and the immune system. Science. 2012;336:1268–73.

105. Andoh A, Imaeda H, Aomatsu T, et al. Comparison of the fecal microbiota profiles between ulcerative colitis and Crohn's disease using terminal restriction fragment length polymorphism analysis. J Gastroenterol. 2011;46:479–86.
106. Ringel-Kulka T, Cheng J, Ringel Y, et al. Intestinal microbiota in healthy U.S. young children and adults – a high throughput microarray analysis. PLoS One. 2013;8(5):e64315. doi:10.1371/journal.pone.0064315.
107. Frank DN, St Amand AL, Feldman RA, Boedeker EC, Harpaz N, Pace NR. Molecular-phylogenetic characterization of microbial community imbalances in human inflammatory bowel diseases. Proc Natl Acad Sci U S A. 2007;104:13780–5.

Chapter 3
Genetics

Akira Meguro and Nobuhisa Mizuki

Abstract The etiology of Behçet's disease (BD) is still unclear, but currently some external environmental factors are thought to trigger BD in individuals with a particular genetic background. It is well established that BD is strongly associated with the human leukocyte antigen (HLA) class I allele, *HLA-B*51*, in many different ethnic groups, indicating that the *HLA-B*51* allele is one of the genetic factors underlying BD. However, the presence of *HLA-B*51*-negative BD patients suggests that other genetic and/or environmental factors also play important roles in the development of BD. Several genes have been recently identified as susceptibility factors for the development of BD, especially with the help of genome-wide association studies. Those findings provide new insights into the genetic tendency underlying BD by connecting classically known findings and allow for clearer interpretation of the etiology and pathophysiology of BD at the molecular level. Thus, findings from genetic studies can provide useful clinical information and open the door to the development of more accurate and reliable diagnostic and treatment approaches for BD.

Keywords Behçet's disease • *HLA-B*51* • Genome-wide association study

3.1 Introduction

Although the etiology of Behçet's disease (BD) is still unclear, genetic and environmental factors likely both play an important role in the development of BD as in many other inflammatory and/or immune-centered diseases. It is well established that the human leukocyte antigen (HLA) class I allele, *HLA-B*51*, is strongly associated with BD. This association indicates that the *HLA-B*51* allele is one of the genetic factors underlying BD. Still, the presence of *HLA-B*51*-negative BD patients suggests that other genetic factors and/or various environmental or infectious agents might also be risk factors for the development of BD. With recent great

A. Meguro (✉) • N. Mizuki
Department of Ophthalmology and Visual Science, Yokohama City University Graduate School of Medicine, 3-9 Fukuura, Kanazawa-ku, Yokohama, Kanagawa 236-0004, Japan
e-mail: akmeguro@yokohama-cu.ac.jp

Y. Ishigatsubo (ed.), *Behçet's Disease*,
DOI 10.1007/978-4-431-54487-6_3

advances in genetic analysis technology, novel candidate genes for BD have recently been identified. This chapter describes classically known and recent genetic findings, as well as their possible involvement in the pathogenesis of BD.

3.2 *HLA-B*51*

HLA, which is the major histocompatibility complex in humans, is located in 6p21.3 on the short arm of chromosome 6. HLA encodes genes involved in antigen processing and the presentation of antigenic peptides to T cells and is instrumental in many innate and adaptive immune responses. Peptide binding to HLA molecules is the single most selective step in the recognition of pathogens by the adaptive immune system and depends on specific amino acids in the peptide-binding groove of each HLA allele. The major special feature of HLA genes is their highest degree of allelic polymorphism in the human genome, and the feature may contribute to individual differences in immune response leading to individual differences in the disease susceptibility.

The strong association between BD and the HLA class I molecule *HLA-B*51* has been well established in many different ethnic groups (Table 3.1) [12–15]. Thus, the *HLA-B*51* allele is the major genetic factor for BD, and the HLA region as a core issue of the *HLA-B* gene has been widely studied in BD. The HLA class I molecules bind peptides from exogenous antigens and present them to CD8+ cells. Peptide binding to HLA is allele specific and depends on the amino acids constituting the peptide-binding groove of each HLA allele. Therefore, immune response to certain peptides varies drastically based on the type of HLA allele possessed and disease

Table 3.1 The HLA-B*51-positive frequencies in Behçet's disease (BD) patients and healthy controls

Country/ethnic group	BD patients (%)	Controls (%)
East Asia		
Japan [1]	58.9	13.8
Korea [2]	35.2	22.5
Middle East		
Iran [3]	61.9	28.7
Jordan [4]	63.2	16.0
Saudi Arabia [5]	76.9	22.2
Turkey [6]	75.0	24.7
Europe		
Italy [7]	57.4	19.2
Spain [8]	36.2	19.6
Greece [9]	78.9	22.5
Germany [6]	57.6	12.3
Caucasian [10]	42.9	10.0

Modified from reference [11]

susceptibility varies among individuals. The frequency of the HLA-B51 antigen is known to be markedly increased in BD patients of many ethnic groups whereas the HLA-B52 antigen, which is identical to HLA-B51 except for two amino acid residues, is not associated with BD. In short, immune response against the specific peptides that bind to these two HLA-B51-specific amino acids may be directly associated with BD development [16]. Peptide-binding motifs of HLA-B51 have in fact been clarified (http://www.syfpeithi.de/); however, exogenous and/or endogenous peptide antigens for BD remain unclear, and thus further studies for them are needed to clarify the HLA-B51-driven immune response in the pathogenesis of BD.

BD exists worldwide but is more prevalent in countries along the Silk Route, between latitudes 30° and 45° north, from the East Asia to the Middle East and the Mediterranean basin [13, 17]. *HLA-B*51* is the most strongly associated with the risk factor for BD in these areas [13, 14]. The prevalences of BD in the Silk Route areas are 10–420 cases per 100,000 individuals, whereas those in Western and Northern Europe and United States (USA) are rare, accounting for less than 1 case per 100,000 individuals [17–19]. The *HLA-B*51* allele-positive frequency in the general European and US populations appears to be low compared with those in the areas along the Silk Route, suggesting that the difference of *HLA-B*51* frequency among these areas reflects regional differences in BD prevalence. On the other hand, the *HLA-B*51*-positive frequencies in Italian, Portuguese, and Eskimo are similar to that in areas along the Silk Route; however, the BD prevalences in Italian and Portuguese are only about 2 cases per 100,000 individuals, and the Eskimo indicates undocumented BD development [17]. This implies that other factors besides *HLA-B*51* seem to be implicated in the development of BD. In addition, BD has never been reported in US-residing Japanese-Americans who share a similar genetic background as native Japanese, in whom the prevalence of BD is 13.5 cases per 100,000 individuals [17, 20, 21]. This fact suggests that certain exogenous factors in the Silk Route areas are involved in the development of BD.

More recently, Hughes et al. performed dense genotyping in the HLA region to locate the genetic association between *HLA-B*51* and BD [22]. They have shown that the genetic association between *HLA-B*51* and BD disappears completely in Turkish and Italian populations after controlling for the effect of rs116799036 (which is located in the approximately 24-kb upstream promoter region of HLA-B). Therefore, they have suggested that the risk ascribed to *HLA-B*51* is likely not causal with respect to BD. Further analysis is required to confirm their findings, with due consideration given to the extensive genetic diversity and the strong linkage disequilibrium in the HLA region.

3.3 Recent Genetic Findings

The *HLA-B*51* allele is the major susceptibility gene responsible for BD. In many ethnic groups, approximately 40–80 % of BD patients possess the *HLA-B*51* allele (Table 3.1) [14]. Hence, about 20–60 % of BD patients lack the *HLA-B*51* allele, suggesting that other genetic factors might also play important roles in the development of BD. To identify novel BD susceptibility genes, "candidate gene analysis" using genes is selected based on symptoms and dysfunctions observed in the disease and "genome-wide association study (GWAS)" using genetic markers across the entire genome have recently been performed. The following are disease-susceptibility genes which have been reported as risk factors for BD.

3.3.1 Candidate Gene Analysis

3.3.1.1 *ICAM1*

Intercellular adhesion molecule-1 (ICAM-1), a cell-adhesion molecule regulating cell-cell interactions in the immunosystem, is mainly expressed on endothelial cells. ICAM-1 expression increases during inflammation, and elevated serum levels of soluble ICAM-1 are observed in patients with inflammatory diseases including BD. Recent studies have reported that the *ICAM1* gene polymorphisms are significantly associated with BD [23, 24].

3.3.1.2 Factor V

BD is a systemic inflammatory disease with high risk of venous thrombosis. Venous thrombosis is the formation of a thrombus within a vein, and BD confers a 14-fold risk of developing venous thrombosis [25]. Since a point mutation (factor V Leiden) in the factor V gene was reported to be associated with thrombophilia [26], factor V Leiden has been focused as a risk factor for venous thrombosis and reported to increase the risk of venous thrombosis in BD [27, 28]. Furthermore, factor V Leiden is significantly associated with ocular involvement in BD [29, 30], thus suggesting the effect on the visual prognosis in BD patients. However, factor V Leiden has not been detected in the Japanese populations [31–33], and this mutation may therefore not be related to the risk of venous thrombosis in Japanese BD patients.

3.3.1.3 *eNOS*

Nitric oxide (NO), which is mainly produced in endothelial cells, contributes to vascular dilatation, inhibition of platelet agglutination and cell-adhesion molecule expression, and vascular smooth muscle relaxation. NO is synthesized from L-arginine by NO synthase (NOS). Three NOS isoforms have been identified: NOS1 (neuronal NOS), NOS2 (inducible NOS), and NOS3 (endothelial NOS: eNOS). Recent studies have demonstrated that the polymorphism in the *eNOS* gene, which is located in the endothelial cells and contributes to leukocyte adhesion inhibition and vascular dilation, is significantly associated with BD [34, 35]. NO level has been reported to decrease in BD patients particularly during the active phase of the disease, and the decreased NO level may be associated with *eNOS* gene polymorphisms and play a crucial role in endothelial dysfunction and thrombosis in BD patients.

3.3.2 Genome-Wide Association Study Findings

A genome-wide association study (GWAS) is an approach that involves rapidly genotyping a dense panel of genetic markers that covers the entire genome and has great power to detect genetic variants that contribute to the risk of developing common and complex diseases. BD susceptibility genes/loci that have been successfully identified by GWASs include *HLA-A*26*, *UBAC2*, *IL10*, *IL23R-IL12RB2*, *STAT4*, *ERAP1*, and *CCR1-CCR3* (Table 3.2).

3.3.2.1 *HLA-A*26*

A GWAS of BD using a Japanese population that employed 23,465 microsatellite markers was published in 2009 [36]. This GWAS identified one marker in the HLA class I region that is not in linkage disequilibrium with *HLA-B*51*. A comprehensive analysis of the HLA class I region found that the *HLA-A*26* allele was significantly associated with BD independently of *HLA-B*51*, suggesting that *HLA-A*26* is the second major susceptibility allele for BD. Individuals with *HLA-B*51*, *HLA-A*26*, or both account for approximately 80 % of all BD patients in Japan. The association of BD with *HLA-A*26* has also been reported in Taiwan, Greece, and Korea [37–39]. In addition, it has been reported that the phenotype frequency of

Table 3.2 Susceptibility genes/loci for Behçet's disease identified by genome-wide association studies

Genes/loci	Ethnic groups[a]
*HLA-A*26*	Japanese [36], Taiwanese [37], Greek [38], Korean [39]
UBAC2	Turk [40, 41], Italian [41], Chinese [42]
IL10	Japanese [43, 44], Turk [43, 44], Korean [44], UK Caucasian [45], Jordanian [45], Palestinian [45], Iranian [46]
IL23R-IL12RB2	Japanese [43, 44], Turk [43, 44], Chinese [47], Iranian [46]
ERAP1	Turk [48]
STAT4	Turk [48], Japanese [48], Chinese [49], Korean [50]
CCR1-CCR3	Turk [48], Japanese [48], Chinese [51]
KLRC4	Turk [48], Japanese [48]
GIMAP	Korean [52], Japanese [52]

Modified from reference [53]
[a]Ethnic groups in which an association was found were listed

*HLA-A*26* was increased ~7-fold in Saudi Arabian patients compared with healthy controls; however, this difference was not statistically significant [5]. Moreover, it has been suggested that *HLA-A*2601*, one of the major *HLA-A*26* subtypes, might be associated with ocular BD in the Japanese population and might also be a marker for poor visual prognosis [54]. In a Korean population study, *HLA-A*2601* and two other alleles (*HLA-A*0207* and *HLA-A*3004*) were significantly associated with an increased risk of developing BD, and *HLA-A*2601* was associated with uveitis; *HLA-A*0207* was associated with skin lesions and arthritis; and *HLA-A*3004* was associated with vascular lesions, genital ulcers, and a positive pathergy test, suggesting that certain *HLA-A* alleles are responsible for the unique clinical features of BD [39]. *HLA-A*26* was not associated with BD in Palestine, Jordan, Iran, Ireland, Italy, or Turkey [55–59], although Remmers et al. [43] have reported a strong association between the HLA-A region and BD independent of *HLA-B*51* in a Turkish population.

There are at least four possible reasons why this association has not been observed in all populations. The first reason is that the frequency of the *HLA-A*26* allele differs among ethnicities. It is more common in Japan, Taiwan, and Korea than in other areas; therefore, the association between *HLA-A*26* and BD may have been easily observed in these countries. Actually, Hughes et al. [22] reported the low allele frequency of *HLA-A*26* in Turkish and Italian populations, in which the association with BD cannot be assessed, while a strong association was observed for *HLA-A*0201*. Second, there have been differences between studies regarding sample size and research strategy. Previous studies with negative results in *HLA-A*26* did not recruit enough samples to provide statistically significant results; they also did not stratify the study population according to *HLA-B*51* status. Third, the environmental factors required for the development of BD associated with the *HLA-A*26* are distributed unevenly throughout the planet. Finally, other genetic factors are highly important in the development of BD in populations in which no association has been observed between *HLA-A*26* and BD. Thus, the association between BD and *HLA-A*26* has not clearly been verified, and further studies are needed to assess the association of BD with *HLA-A*26*.

3.3.2.2 *UBAC2*

A GWAS of BD by Fei et al. in 2009 [40] that employed a dense panel of single-nucleotide polymorphism (SNP) markers reported the five genes *LOC100129342*, *KIAA1529*, *CPVL* (carboxypeptidase, vitellogenic-like), *UBASH3B* (ubiquitin-associated and SH3 domain-containing B), and *UBAC2* (UBA domain-containing 2) in a Turkish population. Of these five, the association of *UBAC2* with the disease has been replicated in other studies [41, 42]. Sawalha et al. found the association of an intronic polymorphism (rs7999348) in Turkish and Italian populations and demonstrated that the expression of *UBAC2* mRNA was significantly increased in the presence of the homozygous risk genotype in rs7999348 [41]. On the other hand, Hou et al. showed the association of a promoter polymorphism (rs3825427) in a

Chinese population and found that the risk allele of rs3825427 significantly down-regulated the expression of *UBAC2* mRNA [42].

UBAC2 encodes an ubiquitination-related structural domain which is implicated in ubiquitination and proteasomal degradation. Other ubiquitination-related genes, *UBASH3B* [40], *SUMO4* (small ubiquitin-like modifier 4) [60–62], and UBE2QL1 (ubiquitin-conjugating enzyme E2Q family-like 1) [43], have also been shown to be associated with BD, suggesting that ubiquitination-related pathway might be involved in the pathogenesis of BD.

3.3.2.3 *IL10* and *IL23R-IL12RB2*

In 2010, two SNP GWASs by Remmers et al. [43] and Mizuki et al. [44] reported the genes that encoded IL-10 (*IL10*), IL-23 receptor (*IL23R*), and IL-12 receptor beta (*IL12B2*) as novel BD susceptibility loci and demonstrated that polymorphisms in these loci are associated with the risk of BD in Turkish, Japanese, and Korean populations. The association of BD with *IL10* polymorphisms has also been reported in Iranian, UK, Jordanian, and Palestinian populations [45, 46], while the association of BD with *IL23R* polymorphisms has also been observed in Chinese populations [47]. In addition, in an Iranian population, *IL23R* and *IL12RB2* polymorphisms were significantly associated with BD, and the importance of *IL23R* regulatory regions has been highlighted with respect to susceptibility to BD [46]. Therefore, it is highly possible that an immune response involving *IL10* and *IL23R* (or *IL12RB2*) contributes to the development of BD.

As *IL10* polymorphisms are associated with decreased *IL10* mRNA expression, it is suggested that decreased expression of IL-10, which downregulates Th1-type immune responses [63, 64], is related to the development of BD. *IL12RB2*, encoding an IL-12 receptor chain, is expressed on Th1 and natural killer (NK) cells [65, 66]. *IL12RB2* polymorphisms might enhance irritability against IL-12, leading to excessive Th1 immune responses. Thus, the activation of a Th1 immune response derived from *IL10* and *IL12RB2* polymorphisms might be involved in BD development.

IL23R encodes a subunit of the IL-23 receptor. *IL23R* is expressed on Th17 cells and macrophages. Recent studies have suggested that Th17 cells are closely correlated with clearance of extracellular bacterial infection, neutrophil chemotaxis, and autoimmune disease development [67–69]. In BD patients, immune response and protection against infections with certain streptococci such as *Streptococcus sanguinis* are enhanced, suggesting that these bacterial infections may serve as triggers for the disease development [70]. As a result, it is suggested that excessive migration of neutrophils into the disease lesions is induced by enhanced neutrophil functions, contributing to the pathogenesis of BD. *IL23R* polymorphisms might enhance irritability to IL-23 in Th17 cells, and accordingly, the Th17 cell-mediated immune response is suggested to be activated and promote BD development.

Summing up, in BD, certain exogenous antigens first induce the immune response via HLA-B51 and HLA-A26 molecules, and subsequently, activation of

Th1 and Th17 immune responses is promoted due to abnormalities of IL-10-regulating Th1 system, IL-12 receptor on Th1 cells, and/or IL-23 receptor on Th17 cells. The result is the chronic inflammation observed in BD patients.

3.3.2.4 *STAT4*

Two SNP GWASs (by Hou et al. in 2012 [49] and Kirino et al. in 2013 [48]) identified the *STAT4* (signal transducer and activator of transcription 4) gene as a susceptibility gene for BD and demonstrated that *STAT4* polymorphisms are associated with the risk of BD in Turkish, Japanese, and Chinese populations. A study in a Korean population has also reported the association of intestinal BD with a *STAT4* polymorphism [50]. In addition, the study also reported that polymorphisms in *IL17A* and *IL23R* were associated with intestinal BD and that gene-gene interactions were observed between *IL17A*, *IL23R*, and *STAT4* polymorphisms, suggesting that the joint effect of SNPs in *IL17A*, *IL23R*, and *STAT4* genes may modulate susceptibility to intestinal BD.

STAT4 encodes a transcription factor that transmits signals induced by several key cytokines, including IL-12 and IL-23 [71]. STAT4 is an essential element in the early events of Th1 differentiation [72]. *STAT4* has also been implicated in the production of IL-17 by the IL-23-differentiated cells, suggesting that it may be involved in the survival or maintenance of Th17 cells [73]. *STAT4* mRNA expression is reportedly higher in individuals with the BD-associated alleles (A alleles of rs7574070 and rs7572482) than in individuals lacking these alleles in a European population [48]. Since both IL-12 and IL-23 act through STAT4, the BD-associated *STAT4* alleles may induce upregulated IL-12 and IL-23 activity, which can lead to the development of BD. In a Chinese population, a BD-associated *STAT4* allele (the A allele of rs897200) was also associated with the upregulation of *STAT4* and the transcription and protein expression of IL-17 (a Th17 cytokine), but not interferon γ (a Th1 cytokine) [49]. These findings suggest that the A allele of rs897200 in *STAT4* might contribute to the pathogenesis of BD through the Th17 pathway, but not the Th1 pathway.

3.3.2.5 *ERAP1*

The endoplasmic reticulum aminopeptidase 1 (*ERAP1*) is centrally involved in peptide trimming before HLA class I presentation. Previous GWASs have shown that *ERAP1* polymorphisms are associated with psoriasis and ankylosing spondylitis [74–76]. There is evidence for gene-gene interactions between *ERAP1* polymorphisms and the disease-associated HLA alleles in both diseases [75, 77]: *ERAP1* polymorphisms affected psoriasis and ankylosing spondylitis susceptibility only in individuals carrying *HLA-C*06* and *HLA-B*27*, respectively.

The SNP GWAS by Kirino et al. in 2013 [48] revealed that *ERAP1* polymorphisms are associated with BD in Turkish populations. The study also identified evidence of an interaction between *HLA-B*51* and *ERAP1* (Fig. 3.1): *ERAP1*

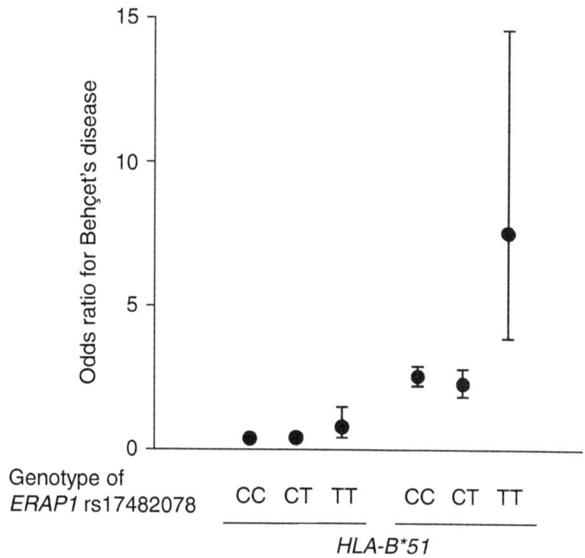

Fig. 3.1 Epistasis between *HLA-B*51* and *ERAP1* rs17482078 in Behçet's disease (Modified from reference [48])

variants affected the risk for BD only in *HLA-B*51*-positive individuals, and homozygosity for the risk allele T at the *ERAP1* locus rs17482078 was associated with an OR for BD of 3.78 among *HLA-B*51*-positive individuals and an OR of 1.48 among *HLA-B*51*-negative individuals. These findings indicate that the BD-associated *ERAP1* variant contributes to disease susceptibility through an interaction with the *HLA-B*51* protein and that modulation of *ERAP1* may be effective in treating BD, especially in *HLA-B*51*-positive patients.

3.3.2.6 *CCR1-CCR3*

The SNP GWAS by Kirino et al. in 2013 [48] also identified BD-associated polymorphisms in the *CCR1* (chemokine (C-C motif) receptor 1)-*CCR3* region in Turkish and Japanese populations. Strong association signals were located in the 3′ untranslated region (UTR) of *CCR1*. The strongest, rs7616215, is located within DNase I hypersensitivity and histone 3 lysine 4 methylation sites, suggesting that the polymorphisms have an effect on transcription. The study actually demonstrated a significant correlation between the disease risk T allele of rs7616215 and enhanced expression of *CCR1* mRNA, but not *CCR3* mRNA. In addition, the study also found that the migration of monocytes in response to a gradient of the CCR1 ligand MIP1-α was less pronounced in T allele-positive individuals than in T allele-negative individuals and that *CCR1* mRNA expression correlated significantly with the chemotactic activity of monocytes against a gradient of MIP1-α. Therefore, the study results suggest that impaired clearance of pathogens may contribute to the etiology of BD. Hou et al. reported that the *CCR1-CCR3* polymorphisms were also associated with BD in a Chinese population: rs13084057 in the 3′ UTR of *CCR1* and rs13075270 and rs13092160 in the intergenic region between *CCR1* and *CCR3* (the 5′ UTR of *CCR1* or the 5′ UTR of *CCR3*) [51]. The study demonstrated that *CCR1* and *CCR3* mRNA expression were reduced in individuals with the TT genotype of rs13092160 (homozygosity for the risk allele), compared with those carrying the CT genotype (heterozygosity for the risk allele), suggesting that both *CCR1* and *CCR3* genes may contribute to the development of BD.

CCR1 and *CCR3* encode the beta chemokine receptor family, which belongs to the G protein-coupled receptor super family. These receptors play an important role in the recruitment and activation of inflammatory cells and contribute to autoimmune and allergic diseases [78, 79]. They are closely located in chromosome 3p21.3 and are considered to have originated from a common ancestral gene, suggesting that the expression of these genes may be regulated through similar pathways [80, 81]. Further investigation is needed to clarify the significance of *CCR1* and *CCR3* in the etiology of BD.

3.4 Summary

We have summarized the susceptibility genes of BD with recent findings to date in this chapter. In addition to the genes discussed above, the *KLRK1* (killer cell lectin-like receptor subfamily K, member 1)-*KLRC4* (killer cell lectin-like receptor subfamily C, member 4) locus on chromosome 12p13.2-p12.3 [48] and the *GIMAP* (GTPases of immunity-associated protein) locus on chromosome 7q36.1 [52] have been identified by GWASs and might also be important for the development of BD. Furthermore, recent deep resequencing analysis of possible candidate genes in BD has identified BD-associated rare and low-frequency non-synonymous variants in the *MEFV* (Mediterranean fever) and *TLR4* (toll-like receptor 4) genes [82], suggesting that these genes play key roles in innate immune and bacterial sensing mechanisms in BD pathogenesis. Thanks to recent great advances in genetic analysis technology, we can now interpret the etiology and pathophysiology of many diseases at genetic level more clearly and rapidly. The final objective of identifying the susceptibility genes for diseases including BD is to apply the new-found knowledge and information in the clinical field, that is to say, not only understanding diseases with genetic findings but also taking a further step forward in clinical medicine to formulate more accurate and reliable diagnosis and treatment of diseases.

References

1. Mizuki N, Ota M, Katsuyama Y, et al. Association analysis between the MIC-A and HLA-B alleles in Japanese patients with Behcet's disease. Arthritis Rheum. 1999;42:1961–6.
2. Park S, Park K, Seo Y, et al. Association of MICA polymorphism with HLA-B51 and disease severity in Korean patients with Behcet's disease. J Korean Med Sci. 2002;17:366–70.

3. Mizuki N, Yabuki K, Ota M, et al. Analysis of microsatellite polymorphism around the HLA-B locus in Iranian patients with Behcet's disease. Tissue Antigens. 2002;60:396–9.
4. Mizuki N, Yabuki K, Ota M, et al. Microsatellite mapping of a susceptible locus within the HLA region for Behcet's disease using Jordanian patients. Hum Immunol. 2001;62:186–90.
5. Yabuki K, Ohno S, Mizuki N, et al. HLA class I and II typing of the patients with Behçet's disease in Saudi Arabia. Tissue Antigens. 1999;54:273–7.
6. Kotter I, Gunaydin I, Stubiger N, et al. Comparative analysis of the association of HLA-B*51 suballeles with Behcet's disease in patients of German and Turkish origin. Tissue Antigens. 2001;58:166–70.
7. Salvarani C, Boiardi L, Mantovani V, et al. Association of MICA alleles and HLA-B51 in Italian patients with Behcet's disease. J Rheumatol. 2001;28:1867–70.
8. Gonzalez-Escribano MF, Rodriguez MR, Aguilar F, et al. Lack association of MICA transmembrane region polymorphism and Behcet's disease in Spain. Tissue Antigens. 1999;54:278–81.
9. Yabuki K, Mizuki N, Ota M, et al. Association of MICA gene and HLA-B*5101 with Behcet's disease in Greece. Invest Ophthalmol Vis Sci. 1999;40:1921–6.
10. Hughes EH, Collins RWM, Kondeatis E, et al. Associations of major histocompatibility complex class I chain-related molecule polymorphisms with Behcet's disease in Caucasian patients. Tissue Antigens. 2005;66:195–9.
11. Meguro A, Mizuki N. HLA and Behçet disease (written in Japanese). J Eye, vol 23. Tokyo: Medical-Aoi Publications; 2006. p. 1521–27.
12. Ono S, Aoki K, Sugiura S, et al. Letter: HL-A5 and Behçet's disease. Lancet. 1973;2:1383–4.
13. Ohno S, Ohguchi M, Hirose S, et al. Close association of HLA-Bw51 with Behçet's disease. Arch Ophthalmol. 1982;100:1455–8.
14. de Menthon M, Lavalley MP, Maldini C, et al. HLA-B51/B5 and the risk of Behçet's disease: a systematic review and meta-analysis of case–control genetic association studies. Arthritis Rheum. 2009;61:1287–96.
15. Gul A, Ohno S. HLA-B*51 and Behçet disease. Ocul Immunol Inflamm. 2012;20:37–43.
16. Mizuki N, Inoko H, Mizuki N, et al. Human leukocyte antigen serologic and DNA typing of Behçet's disease and its primary association with B51. Invest Ophthalmol Vis Sci. 1992;33:3332–40.
17. Verity DH, Marr JE, Ohno S, et al. Behçet's disease, the Silk Road and HLA-B51: historical and geographical perspectives. Tissue Antigens. 1999;54:213–20.
18. Al-Otaibi LM, Porter SR, Poate TWJ. Behçet's disease: a review. J Dent Res. 2005;84:209–22.
19. Azizlerli G, Köse AA, Sarica R, et al. Prevalence of Behcet's disease in Istanbul, Turkey. Int J Dermatol. 2003;42:803–6.
20. Hirohata T, Kuratsune M, Nomura A, et al. Prevalence of Behçet's syndrome in Hawaii, with particular references to the comparison of the Japanese in Hawaii and Japan. Hawaii Med J. 1975;34:244–6.
21. Ohno S, Char DH, Kimura SJ, et al. Clinical observations in Behçet's disease. Jpn J Ophthalmol. 1979;23:126–31.
22. Hughes T, Coit P, Adler A, et al. Identification of multiple independent susceptibility loci in the HLA region in Behçet's disease. Nat Genet. 2013;45:319–24.
23. Verity DH, Vaughan RW, Kondeatis E, et al. Intercellular adhesion molecule-1 gene polymorphisms in Behcet's disease. Eur J Immunogenet. 2000;27:73–6.
24. Boiardi L, Salvarani C, Casali B, et al. Intercellular adhesion molecule-1 gene polymorphisms in Behcet's disease. J Rheumatol. 2001;28:1283–7.
25. Ames PR, Steuer A, Pap A, et al. Thrombosis in Behcet's disease: a retrospective survey from a single UK centre. Rheumatology. 2001;40:652–5.
26. Bertina RM, Koeleman BP, Koster T, et al. Mutation in blood coagulation factor V associated with resistance to activated protein C. Nature. 1994;369:64–7.
27. Gül A, Ozbek U, Oztürk C, et al. Coagulation factor V gene mutation increases the risk of venous thrombosis in Behcet's disease. Br J Rheumatol. 1996;35:1178–80.

28. Mammo L, Al-Dalaan A, Bahabri SS, et al. Association of factor V Leiden with Behcet's disease. J Rheumatol. 1997;24:2196–8.
29. Verity DH, Vaughan RW, Madanat W, et al. Factor V Leiden mutation associated with ocular involvement in Behcet's disease. Am J Ophthalmol. 1999;128:352–6.
30. Batioğlu F, Atmaca LS, Karabulut HG, et al. Factor V Leiden and prothrombin gene G20210A mutations in ocular Behcet's disease. Acta Ophthalmol Scand. 2003;81:283–5.
31. Zama T, Murata M, Ono F, et al. Low prevalence of activated protein C resistance and coagulation factor V Arg506 to Gln mutation among Japanese patients with various forms of thrombosis, and normal individuals. Int J Hematol. 1996;65:71–8.
32. Seki T, Okayama H, Kumagai T, et al. Arg506Gln mutation of the coagulation factor V gene not detected in Japanese pulmonary thromboembolism. Heart Vessel. 1998;13:195–8.
33. Kobashi G, Yamada H, Asano T, et al. The factor V Leiden mutation is not a common cause of pregnancy-induced hypertension in Japan. Semin Thromb Hemost. 1999;25:487–9.
34. Salvarani C, Boiardi L, Casali B, et al. Endothelial nitric oxide synthase gene polymorphisms in Behçet's disease. J Rheumatol. 2002;29:535–40.
35. Karasneh JA, Hajeer AH, Silman A, et al. Polymorphisms in the endothelial nitric oxide synthase gene are associated with Behcet's disease. Rheumatology. 2005;44:614–17.
36. Meguro A, Inoko H, Ota M, et al. Genetics of Behçet's disease inside and outside the MHC. Ann Rheum Dis. 2010;69:747–54.
37. Chung YM, Yeh TS, Sheu MM, et al. Behcet's disease with ocular involvement in Taiwan: a joint survey of six major ophthalmological departments. J Formos Med Assoc. 1990;89:413–17.
38. Mizuki N, Ohno S, Ando H, et al. A strong association between HLA-B*5101 and Behçet's disease in Greek patients. Tissue Antigens. 1997;50:57–60.
39. Kang EH, Kim JY, Takeuchi F, et al. Associations between the HLA-A polymorphism and the clinical manifestations of Behcet's disease. Arthritis Res Ther. 2011;13:R49.
40. Fei Y, Webb R, Cobb BL, et al. Identification of novel genetic susceptibility loci for Behçet's disease using a genome-wide association study. Arthritis Res Ther. 2009;11:R66.
41. Sawalha AH, Hughes T, Nadig A, et al. A putative functional variant within the UBAC2 gene is associated with increased risk of Behçet's disease. Arthritis Rheum. 2011;63:3607–12.
42. Hou S, Shu Q, Jiang Z, et al. Replication study confirms the association between UBAC2 and Behçet's disease in two independent Chinese sets of patients and controls. Arthritis Res Ther. 2012;14:R70.
43. Remmers EF, Cosan F, Kirino Y, et al. Genome-wide association study identifies variants in the MHC class I, IL10, and IL23R-IL12RB2 regions associated with Behçet's disease. Nat Genet. 2010;42:698–702.
44. Mizuki N, Meguro A, Ota M, et al. Genome-wide association studies identify IL23R-IL12RB2 and IL10 as Behçet's disease susceptibility loci. Nat Genet. 2010;42:703–6.
45. Wallace GR, Kondeatis E, Vaughan RW, et al. IL-10 genotype analysis in patients with Behçet's disease. Hum Immunol. 2007;68:122–7.
46. Xavier JM, Shahram F, Davatchi F, et al. Association study of IL10 and IL23R-IL12RB2 in Iranian patients with Behçet's disease. Arthritis Rheum. 2012;64:2761–72.
47. Jiang Z, Yang P, Hou S, et al. IL-23R gene confers susceptibility to Behcet's disease in a Chinese Han population. Ann Rheum Dis. 2010;69:1325–8.
48. Kirino Y, Bertsias G, Ishigatsubo Y, et al. Genome-wide association analysis identifies new susceptibility loci for Behçet's disease and epistasis between HLA-B*51 and ERAP1. Nat Genet. 2013;45:202–7.
49. Hou S, Yang Z, Du L, et al. Identification of a susceptibility locus in STAT4 for Behçet's disease in Han Chinese in a genome-wide association study. Arthritis Rheum. 2012;64:4104–13.
50. Kim ES, Kim SW, Moon CM, et al. Interactions between IL17A, IL23R, and STAT4 polymorphisms confer susceptibility to intestinal Behcet's disease in Korean population. Life Sci. 2012;90:740–6.
51. Hou S, Xiao X, Li F, et al. Two-stage association study in Chinese Han identifies two independent associations in CCR1/CCR3 locus as candidate for Behçet's disease susceptibility. Hum Genet. 2012;131:1841–50.

52. Lee YJ, Horie Y, Wallace GR, et al. Genome-wide association study identifies GIMAP as a novel susceptibility locus for Behcet's disease. Ann Rheum Dis. 2013;72(9):1510–16. doi:10.1136/annrheumdis-2011-200288.
53. Meguro A, Inoko H. Genetic factors of Behçet disease (written in Japanese). Inflamm Immun, vol 21. Tokyo: Sentan Igaku-sya; 2013. p. 17–23.
54. Kaburaki T, Takamoto M, Numaga J, et al. Genetic association of HLA-A*2601 with ocular Behçet's disease in Japanese patients. Clin Exp Rheumatol. 2010;28:S39–44.
55. Verity DH, Wallace GR, Vaughan RW, et al. HLA and tumour necrosis factor (TNF) polymorphisms in ocular Behçet's disease. Tissue Antigens. 1999;54:264–72.
56. Mizuki N, Ota M, Katsuyama Y, et al. HLA class I genotyping including HLA-B*51 allele typing in the Iranian patients with Behçet's disease. Tissue Antigens. 2001;57:457–62.
57. Kilmartin DJ, Finch A, Acheson RW. Primary association of HLA-B51 with Behçet's disease in Ireland. Br J Ophthalmol. 1997;81:649–53.
58. Kera J, Mizuki N, Ota M, et al. Significant associations of HLA-B*5101 and B*5108, and lack of association of class II alleles with Behçet's disease in Italian patients. Tissue Antigens. 1999;54:565–71.
59. Pirim I, Atasoy M, Ikbal M, et al. HLA class I and class II genotyping in patients with Behcet's disease: a regional study of eastern part of Turkey. Tissue Antigens. 2004;64:293–7.
60. Hou S, Yang P, Du L, et al. SUMO4 gene polymorphisms in Chinese Han patients with Behcet's disease. Clin Immunol. 2008;129:170–5.
61. Kamoun M, Ben Dhifallah I, Karray E, et al. Association of small ubiquitin-like modifier 4 (SUMO4) polymorphisms in a Tunisian population with Behçet's disease. Clin Exp Rheumatol. 2010;28:S45–9.
62. Park G, Kim HS, Choe JY, et al. SUMO4 C438T polymorphism is associated with papulopustular skin lesion in Korean patients with Behçet's disease. Rheumatol Int. 2012;32:3031–7.
63. Mosmann TR, Coffman RL, et al. Thl and Th2 cells: different patterns of lymphokine secretion lead to different functional properties. Ann Rev Immunol. 1989;7:145–73.
64. Fiorentino DF, Zlotnik A, Vieira P, et al. IL-10 acts on the antigen presenting cell to inhibit cytokine production by Th1 cells. J Immunol. 1991;146:3444–51.
65. Desai BB, Quinn PM, Wolitzky AG, et al. IL-12 receptor. II. Distribution and regulation of receptor expression. J Immunol. 1992;148:3125–32.
66. Rogge L, Barberis-Maino L, Biffi M, et al. Selective expression of an interleukin-12 receptor component by human T helper 1 cells. J Exp Med. 1997;185:825–31.
67. Iwakura Y, Ishigame H. The IL-23/IL-17 axis in inflammation. J Clin Invest. 2006;116:1218–22.
68. Steinman L. Mixed results with modulation of TH-17 cells in human autoimmune diseases. Nat Immunol. 2009;11:41–4.
69. Khader SA, Gaffen SL, Kolls JK. Th17 cells at the crossroads of innate and adaptive immunity against infectious diseases at the mucosa. Mucosal Immunol. 2009;2:403–11.
70. Isogai E, Ohno S, Kotake S, et al. Chemiluminescence of neutrophils from patients with Behçet's disease and its correlation with an increased proportion of uncommon serotypes of Streptococcus sanguis in the oral flora. Arch Oral Biol. 1990;35:43–8.
71. Watford WT, Hissong BD, Bream JH, et al. Signaling by IL-12 and IL-23 and the immunoregulatory roles of STAT4. Immunol Rev. 2004;202:139–56.
72. Nishikomori R, Usui T, Wu CY, et al. Activated STAT4 has an essential role in Th1 differentiation and proliferation that is independent of its role in the maintenance of IL-12R beta 2 chain expression and signaling. J Immunol. 2002;169:4388–98.
73. Mathur AN, Chang HC, Zisoulis DG, et al. Stat3 and Stat4 direct development of IL-17-secreting Th cells. J Immunol. 2007;178:4901–7.
74. Sun LD, Cheng H, Wang ZX, et al. Association analyses identify six new psoriasis susceptibility loci in the Chinese population. Nat Genet. 2010;42:1005–9.
75. Genetic Analysis of Psoriasis Consortium & the Wellcome Trust Case Control Consortium 2, Strange A, Capon F, et al. A genome-wide association study identifies new psoriasis susceptibility loci and an interaction between HLA-C and ERAP1. Nat Genet. 2010;42:985–90.

76. Wellcome Trust Case Control Consortium, Australo-Anglo-American Spondylitis Consortium (TASC), Burton PR, Clayton DG, et al. Association scan of 14,500 nonsynonymous SNPs in four diseases identifies autoimmunity variants. Nat Genet. 2007;39:1329–37.
77. Evans DM, Spencer CC, Pointon JJ, et al. Interaction between ERAP1 and HLA-B27 in ankylosing spondylitis implicates peptide handling in the mechanism for HLA-B27 in disease susceptibility. Nat Genet. 2011;43:761–7.
78. Diedrichs-Mohring M, Nelson PJ, Proudfoot AE, et al. The effect of the CC chemokine receptor antagonist Met-RANTES on experimental autoimmune uveitis and oral tolerance. J Neuroimmunol. 2005;164:22–30.
79. Nibbs RJB, Salcedo TW, Campbell JDM, et al. C-C chemokine receptor 3 antagonism by the beta-chemokine macrophage inflammatory protein 4, a property strongly enhanced by an amino-terminal alanine-methionine swap. J Immunol. 2000;164:1488–97.
80. Neote K, DiGregorio D, Mak JY, et al. Molecular cloning, functional expression, and signaling characteristics of a C-C chemokine receptor. Cell. 1993;72:415–25.
81. Daugherty BL, Springer MS. The beta-chemokine receptor genes CCR1 (CMKBR1), CCR2 (CMKBR2), and CCR3 (CMKBR3) cluster within 285 kb on human chromosome 3p21. Genomics. 1997;41:294–5.
82. Kirino Y, Zhou Q, Ishigatsubo Y, et al. Targeted resequencing implicates the familial Mediterranean fever gene MEFV and the toll-like receptor 4 gene TLR4 in Behçet disease. Proc Natl Acad Sci U S A. 2013;110:8134–9.

Chapter 4
Ocular Involvement

Toshikatsu Kaburaki

Abstract Ocular involvement in Behçet's disease (BD) is characterized by recurrent explosive attacks of intraocular inflammation, including iridocyclitis, hypopyon, chorioretinitis, retinal vasculitis, retinal vein occlusion, optic neuritis, retinal neovascularization, and vitreous hemorrhage, while uveitis is more common in young males. Retinal disease, especially occlusive retinal vasculitis, is one of the most serious complications and can lead to permanent retinal damage and visual impairment. Colchicine, cyclosporine, corticosteroid, azathioprine, and other immunosuppressive agents are generally used to manage ocular inflammatory attacks. Recently, antitumor necrosis factor-α agents have been shown to dramatically reduce the frequency of ocular attacks in BD patients with refractory uveoretinitis, indicating it as a promising therapy for ocular BD.

Keywords Uveitis • Iridocyclitis • Ocular attack • Retinal vasculitis • Antitumor necrosis factor-α agents

4.1 Introduction

Ocular involvement is one of the most characteristic manifestations of Behçet's disease (BD) and important for diagnosis. Notably, retinal vascular involvement is a common finding in affected patients, which often has devastating effects on eyesight. Visual prognosis for ocular BD patients was extremely poor three decades ago. However, that has been gradually improving especially in recent years, likely due to advancements in immunosuppressive agents.

T. Kaburaki (✉)
Department of Ophthalmology, Graduate School of Medicine, The University of Tokyo, 7-3-1 Hongo, Bunkyo-ku, Tokyo 113-8655, Japan
e-mail: kabutosi-tky@umin.ac.jp

Y. Ishigatsubo (ed.), *Behçet's Disease*,
DOI 10.1007/978-4-431-54487-6_4

4.2 Epidemiology

The frequency of ocular involvement in BD ranges from 30 to 70 %, with differences related to age, sex, and country [1–6]. Ocular symptoms are frequently encountered in young male patients and appear at lower frequency in older females.

In Japan, BD was the most frequent diagnosis (25 %) in uveitis cases in the 1960s [7], after which new-onset patients with ocular BD began to gradually decrease. In a recent multicenter survey held in 2009 in Japan, BD was the 5th most frequent diagnosis (3.9 %) among 3,830 newly arrived uveitis patients in 36 university hospitals [8]. On the other hand, in Turkey, BD remains the most frequent type of uveitis (32 %) among those patients in a multicenter survey [2]. In other countries, the rate of BD in newly arrived patients with uveitis in referral centers or university hospitals was 8.6 % in Iran [9], 7.1 % in southern Thailand [10], 3.5 % in Saudi Arabia [11], 3.1 % in northeastern Italy [12], 1.1 % in Switzerland [13], 0.8 % in California, USA [14], and 0.3 % in India [15].

Four national surveys of BD patients have been performed in Japan, in 1972, 1984, 1991, and 2002. Those showed that the frequency of ocular symptoms in BD is higher in men than women, while the symptoms are gradually decreasing in both genders [6]. In the 2002 survey, ocular symptoms were seen in 72 % of male and 45 % of female patients, and the percentage suffering from uveitis among all BD patients was also gradually decreasing.

Clinical features of uveitis in BD are somewhat different between regions and ethnic groups. The disease is more common and the symptoms more severe in Japanese and Turkish patients [16, 17]. An international survey of the clinical features of 1,465 prevalent cases of ocular BD was performed in 25 eye centers in 14 different countries in 2006 [18]. Intraocular inflammation was bilateral in the majority of patients (85.6 % of women, 85.5 % of men). Recurrence of uveitis was seen in 95.6 % of the women and 95.7 % of the men, while panuveitis, not solely anterior uveitis, was seen more often in men (95.4 %) than in women (89.8 %). Ocular symptoms began younger than 30 years old in most of the countries surveyed, though Japanese patients were the oldest (average 34.3 years old). The percentage of men was significantly higher in India (92 %) than in other countries (57–76 %) [18].

4.3 Clinical Symptoms

The eye is the most commonly involved vital organ in BD and a typical form of involvement is relapsing remitting uveitis. The natural course of the disease is recurrent explosive worsening of intraocular inflammation, the so-called ocular attacks, and spontaneous remission.

Ocular symptoms typically occur within 2–4 years of disease onset in the vast majority of clinical cases [19, 20]. Moreover, ocular disease may be the initial manifestation of the disease in approximately one-fifth of the cases. In general, initial exacerbations tend to be more anterior and unilateral, whereas subsequent attacks tend to involve the vitreous cavity and posterior segment of the eye and gradually become bilateral. In the early period of the disease, slight visual impairment, a few floaters, and eye redness are the major complaints. As the disease progresses, visual impairment and redness gradually become stronger. At the time of an ocular attack, patients usually notice sudden onset of blurred vision, eye pain, photophobia, lacrimation with or without eye redness, floaters, and/or aggravation of visual acuity. The worsening of intraocular inflammation usually continues for one or a few weeks and then spontaneously disappears. Non-permanent, recurrent episodic inflammation is an important characteristic of BD. Ocular disease occurs in 30–70 % of patients with BD (up to 70–90 % in young men) [1–6] and affects both eyes in most patients (about 90 %) during the disease course.

4.3.1 Anterior Involvement

Uveitis in BD has a nongranulomatous characteristic and eventually involves both the anterior and posterior segments of the bilateral eyes in most patients. Major ocular findings observed in BD patients with anterior uveitis are ciliary injection, anterior chamber cells, fine keratic precipitates, and hypopyon, with fibrinous reactions seen in severe cases (Fig. 4.1a–d).

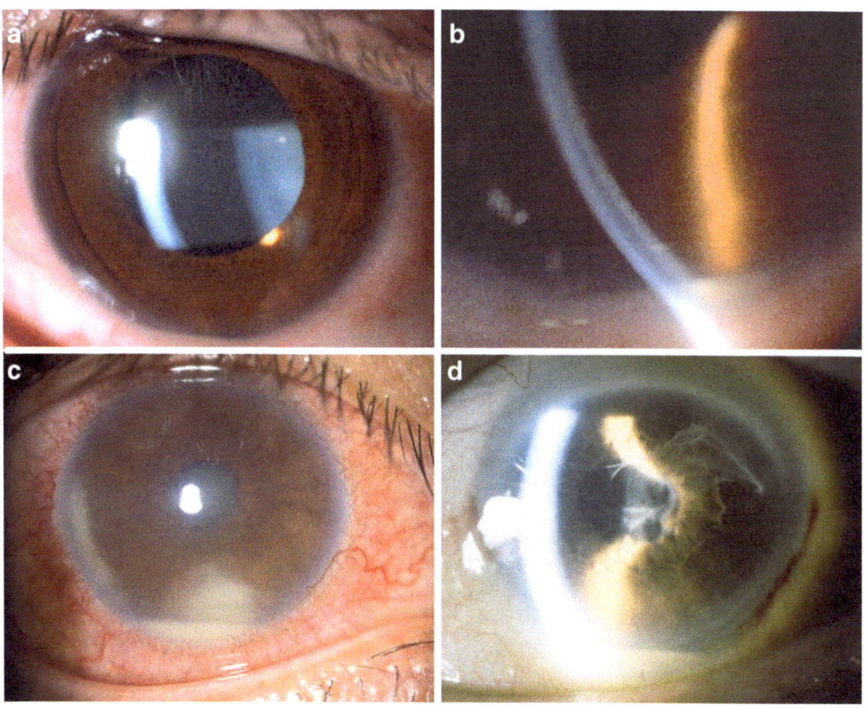

Fig. 4.1 Major ocular findings observed in Behçet's disease patients with anterior uveitis. Ciliary injection (**a**, **c**), anterior chamber cells (**a**, **b**, **d**), fine keratic precipitates (**b**), and hypopyon and/or fibrinous reaction (**b**, **c**, **d**) are commonly seen

The presence of cells (Fig. 4.1a, b, d) in the anterior chamber is the most characteristic finding of an ocular inflammatory attack. These cells may disappear after a while, which indicates the end of the ocular attack. Ciliary injection (Fig. 4.1a, c) is not a constant feature and is found during an ocular inflammatory attack, especially in severe cases. Keratic precipitates (Fig. 4.1b) are also seen during an ocular inflammatory attack, are fine and nonpigmented in most cases, and rarely develop into "mutton-fat" shapes. Confocal microscopy has shown that keratic precipitates in BD are made up of small round cells, one of five types of keratic precipitates identified in ocular inflammatory disease [21].

Hypopyon (Fig. 4.1b, c, d) is sediment formations composed of inflammatory cells in the lower part of the anterior chamber and observed in patients with severe inflammatory attacks. This condition is seen in one-third of ocular BD patients in Japan [7], as compared to 10–35 % of cases in other parts of the world [22, 23]. Small hypopyon can only be seen using a gonioscopic lens, the so-called angle hypopyon. In a Japanese series, macroscopic hypopyon occurred in 12 %, with angle hypopyon visible in 19 % [7]. Hypopyon in BD usually forms a niveau and is not sticky and smoothly moves according to head positioning. On the other hand, a hypopyon in patients with HLA B-27-associated uveitis usually do not show niveau formation, rather a mild elevation in the center of the hypopyon that is mountain-shaped and sticky enough so as to not move according to head positioning. The hypopyon is evanescent and dissolves rapidly even without treatment.

Posterior synechia is found in some patients after anterior uveitis, which remains permanently and sometimes enlarges the area by recurrent anterior uveitis. When synechia occurs along the whole circumference of the pupil, iris bombe may increase intraocular pressure.

4.3.2 Vitritis

Vitritis is another common symptom of ocular attack in BD. Although opacities are often diffuse, a localized snow ball-like vitreous opacity may occasionally be observed. Vitreous haze usually increases during the ocular attack with posterior segment involvement. In severe cases, retinal vessels cannot be seen due to a dense vitreous haze.

4.3.3 Posterior Involvement

Retinal disease is one of the most serious complications and can lead to permanent retinal damage and visual impairment. Various features have been seen in fundus examinations, such as retinal exudates, retinal hemorrhages, perivasculitis, vascular occlusions, retinal edema, and optic disc edema (Fig. 4.2a–d). Retinal exudates are characterized by scattered superficial yellowish white solitary or multifocal

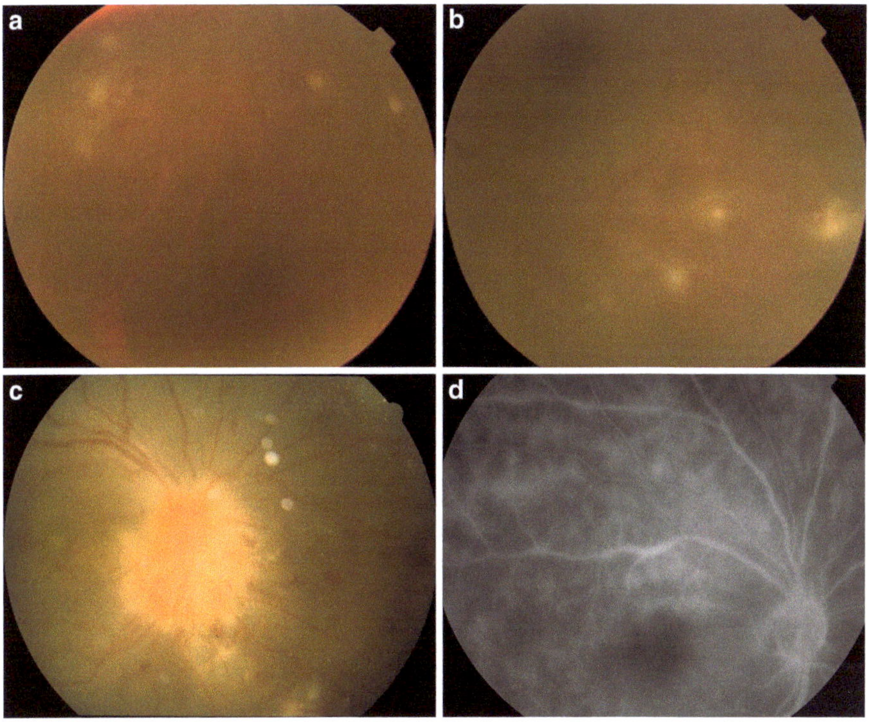

Fig. 4.2 Major ocular findings observed in posterior uveitis in Behçet's disease. Retinal exudates and hemorrhages (**a**), occlusive retinal vasculitis (**b**), massive deep retinal exudates with vascular obliteration (**c**), and massive leakage from retinal capillary vessels, the so-called fern-like leakage (**d**), are often seen

infiltrates of the inner retina and often seen in a posterior ocular attack, usually in the peripheral retina with or without retinal hemorrhages (Fig. 4.2a). Another common finding is occlusive retinal vasculitis (Fig. 4.2b). The retinal vein is predominantly affected (periphlebitis) and the retinal arteries (periarteritis) less frequently. Such lesions are usually transient and heal without scarring, while massive deep retinal exudates involve the outer retinal layers and are associated with vascular obliteration (Fig. 4.2c). This involvement may cause permanent tissue damage of the retina. Branch retinal vein occlusion is rarely seen. Cystoid macular edema (CME) has been reported not only in exacerbation but also convalescent stages. Long-time continuation of chronic CME can cause macular degeneration and permanent visual impairment. Furthermore, severe inflammation of the retina and retinal vascular occlusion can cause neovascularization from the retina and optic disc. The breakdown of neovascular vessels, seen as vitreous hemorrhages, usually occurs recurrently and worsens the clarity of the vitreous.

Fluorescein angiography (FA) is a useful tool for evaluation of the vasculature in the retina and optic disc. Characteristic FA findings in BD are staining and leakage in the optic disc, vascular wall staining due to retinal perivasculitis, and diffuse leakage from retinal vessels and retinal capillary vessels. Notably, massive leakage from retinal capillary vessels, the so-called fern-like leakage (Fig. 4.2d), is a characteristic finding of FA in patients with BD in Japan. It is observed not only during an ocular attack but also in convalescent stages in the majority of patients [24, 25]. However, this finding is not so frequent in Turkish patients (38 %) [26]. Such background leakage from the retina and optic disc was significantly improved in 11 of 14 patients (79 %) after 12 months of infliximab therapy, suggesting that vascular leakage shown by FA serves as an important surrogate marker for the degree of inflammatory control in BD patients receiving various drug regimens [27]. CME, capillary non-perfusion, vascular occlusion, collateral formation, and neovascularization from the retina and optic disc can also be shown by FA. On the other hand, optical coherence tomography (OCT) may be helpful for the detection of an epiretinal membrane, macular hole, CME (Fig. 4.3b), and retinal atrophy.

Multiple recurrent inflammatory attacks of the retina may gradually lead to permanent retinal atrophic changes and the optic disc can also become atrophic. Such damage may parallel the accumulative numbers and severity of posterior ocular attacks [20, 28]. Especially, retinal exudative lesions in the macula and retina around the optic disc may cause damage to the macula and/or optic disc and can lead to a permanent decrease in visual acuity. Recurrent episodes of ocular attack with retinal vasculitis can cause attenuation of retinal vessels, the so-called white vessels. Such retinal damage shows retinal pigment epithelial degeneration, chorioretinal atrophy, macular degeneration, and optic disc atrophy.

4.3.4 Other Ocular Manifestations

Other ocular manifestations of BD include scleritis, episcleritis, filamentary keratitis, conjunctivitis, and subconjunctival hemorrhages. On the other hand, conjunctival ulcerations are rarely seen.

4.4 Complications

Complications from repeated inflammatory attacks are a major concern and depend on where the inflammation is located. Intraocular pressure (IOP) becomes elevated as a result of inflammatory cell plugging of the trabecular meshwork, trabeculitis, advanced posterior synechiae, iris bombe (Fig. 4.3a), peripheral anterior synechiae, neovascular glaucoma, and/or prolonged use of topical or systemic corticosteroids (steroid glaucoma). In large case studies, secondary glaucoma has been found in approximately 11–20 % of ocular BD patients [29, 30]. About half of those cases were steroid- or inflammation-induced open-angle glaucoma, one-fourth were partial angle-closure glaucoma with peripheral anterior synechiae, and one-fifth were angle-closure glaucoma with peripheral anterior synechiae associated with a pupil

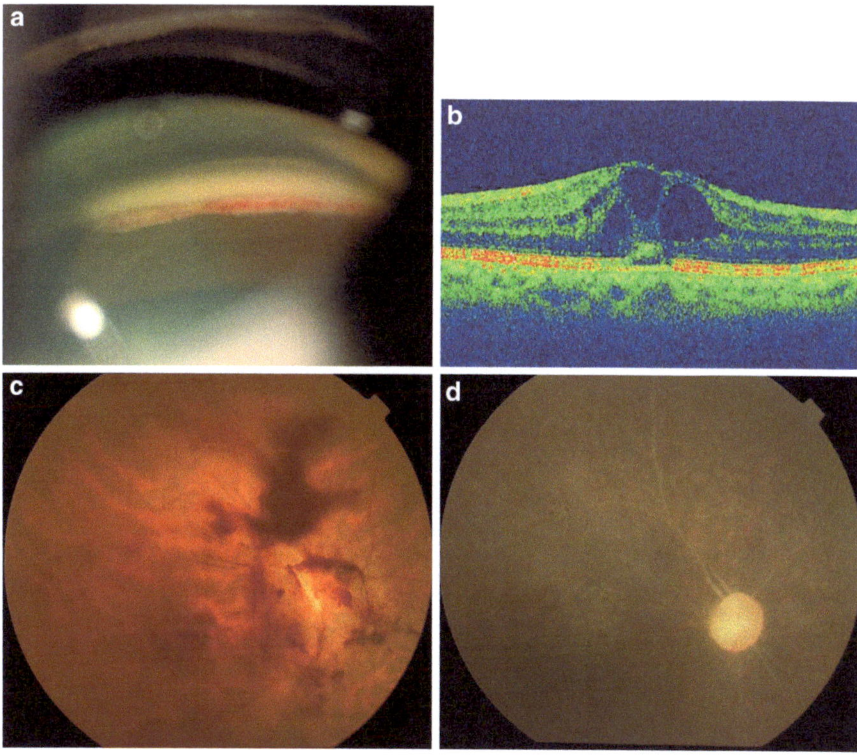

Fig. 4.3 Major complications observed in Behçet's disease. Neovascular glaucoma with angle rubeosis (**a**), cystoid macular edema by optical coherent tomography (**b**), neovascularization of the optic disc (**c**), and sheathing of vessels with retinal and optic disc atrophy (**d**) are often seen

block. The remaining 10 % of the cases suffered from neovascular glaucoma [30]. Cataract formation may also develop due to recurrent ocular attacks during the course of the disease or as a consequence of systemic or topical corticosteroids used for treatment. Most cataracts are posterior subcapsular in location, though anterior subcapsular opacities or a cortical cataract may also be seen.

CME (Fig. 4.3b) is one of the most common complications and observed in 34 % of BD patients [25]. Without appropriate treatment, a chronic CME could progress to permanent macular degeneration with structural changes. Incorporation into the intraretinal cystoid spaces may lead to formation of a partial or full-thickness macular hole in about 10 % of affected cases [31]. An epiretinal membrane is another common complication in BD. Gliotic sheathing of retinal vessels is a typical sequela of retinal periphlebitis. Branch retinal vascular occlusion is occasionally seen in posterior segment inflammatory attacks, while central retinal vascular occlusion is quite rare.

Neovascularization from the optic disc and/or retina (Fig. 4.3c) develops in about 4.3 % of patients and may be associated with retinal ischemia or severe and persistent intraocular inflammation [10, 32]. Such neovascularization from the disc is rather common in cases with frequent ocular attacks and may occur without a non-perfusion area of the retina [32]. Neovascularization from the optic disc and/or retina can often lead to intravitreal hemorrhage and may become a cause of formation of a retinal tear, rhegmatogenous retinal detachment, or tractional retinal detachment. In the final period of the disease, repeated episodes of posterior segment inflammation and complications result in sheathing of vessels due to vascular attenuation and/or sclerosed vessels, diffuse retinal atrophy, and total optic atrophy (Fig. 4.3d), which are typical fundus features of end-stage ocular BD leading to eventual complete blindness.

4.5 Disease Course and Visual Prognoses

Ocular inflammatory attacks with retinal vasculitis can cause retinal damage and permanent visual loss. Notably, repeated retinal exudative lesions and/or hemorrhages in the vascular arcade, which is the region around the macula made up of vessels stemming out from the optic disc, form macular degeneration and optic disc atrophy, resulting in irreversible visual loss. Not only anatomical classification but also the frequency and severity of intraocular inflammation are likely related to visual loss.

The anatomical classification of intraocular inflammation is important for prediction of visual prognoses and therapeutic decisions. Patients with ocular inflammatory exacerbation localized to the anterior segment, the anterior uveitis type, can be treated with corticosteroids as topical treatment and/or a subconjunctival injection. Inflammatory changes usually disappear without permanent tissue damage, despite cataract formation and secondary glaucoma, and visual prognosis in those cases is favorable. On the other hand, patients with inflammatory exacerbation involving the posterior segment, the chorioretinitis type, require systemic treatment for suppression of future ocular inflammatory attacks and to avoid progression of retinal/optic nerve damage.

As for the frequency and severity of ocular attacks, a retrospective study of 39 Japanese BD cases continuously observed for 10 years from the onset of ocular disease was reported [33]. The average number of ocular attacks per eye per year gradually decreased from 4.1 in the first year to 2.2 and 1.4 after 5 and 10 years, respectively [33]. Nevertheless, ocular attacks were still observed in 45 % of those patients even after 10 years from onset, and there was a significant relationship between the accumulative number of ocular attacks and worse visual prognosis [33]. However, in general, there are no further attacks after 15–20 years from onset in most cases [34].

Changes in visual acuity during the disease course of a representative ocular BD patient with recurrent severe chorioretinitis are illustrated in Fig. 4.4. That patient suffered 17 attacks in the right eye and 18 in the left over a 9-year period. During ocular attacks involving the posterior segment of the eyes, visual acuity was decreased. Thereafter, the declined visual acuity recovered with treatment such as

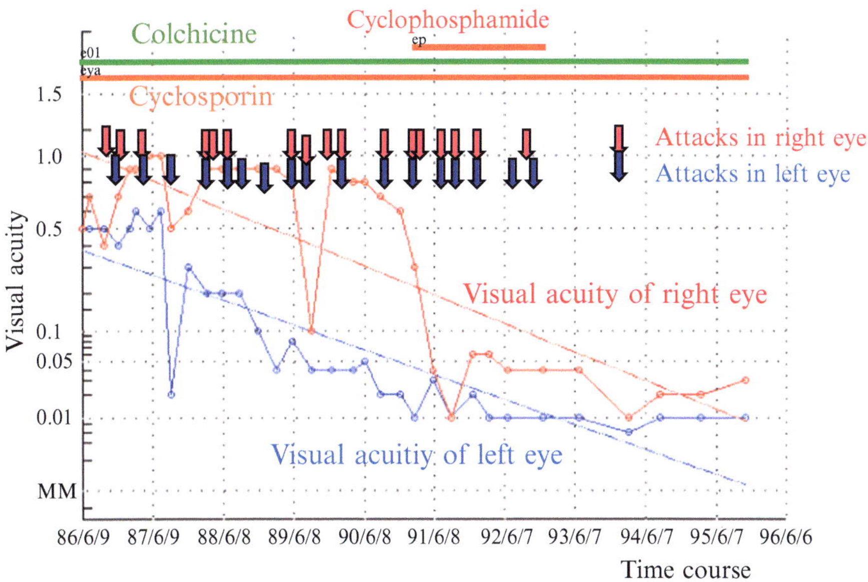

Fig. 4.4 Changing of visual acuity during the clinical course of Behçet's disease with severe recurrent chorioretinitis. This representative patient suffered 17 attacks in the right eye and 18 in the left over a 9-year period. Despite intensive immunosuppressive treatment, frequent severe attacks occurred and the patient lost useful vision in both eyes

subconjunctival corticosteroid injections, at least in the early period of the disease course. However, despite intensive immunosuppressive treatment, severe attacks frequently recurred and the patient lost useful vision in both eyes 5 years after onset. Thus, prevention of recurrent ocular attacks, especially in the posterior segment, is most important for retention of vision.

Many reports have been published about the factors for poor visual prognoses in BD, such as male gender [7, 17, 18, 20, 35], young age [36], higher frequency of ocular attacks [33, 37], chorioretinitis type [7, 20], presence of skin lesions and/or arthritis [20], central nervous system involvement [20, 36], vascular thrombosis [36], strong vitreous opacity and exudates within the retinal arcade [37], current active intraocular inflammation [38], unilateral disease [35], disc neovascularization [25], presence of macular ischemia on fluorescein angiography [25], poor visual acuity at the initial visit [39], and HLA-A26 positivity [40]. On the other hand, female gender [7, 17, 18, 20, 35], anterior uveitis type [7, 20], and the use of biological agents (antitumor necrosis factor (TNF)-α) [35] have been found to be related to retention of vision. There seems to be consensus that the main determinant of visual prognosis is the number of ocular attacks including those in the posterior retina, because they directly induce tissue damage in the macula and/or optic disc. Male sex as a prognostic factor for poor vision has been demonstrated in many reports and confirmed in a recent international survey of ocular BD conducted in 25 eye centers of 14 countries in 2006 [18]. Twenty-three percent of those patients had visual acuity equal to or worse than 20/200 at the final visit, with poor visual acuity seen in 18.9 % of females and 24.8 % of males ($p < 0.01$). Those with poor vision were more frequently seen in India, Iran, and Japan than the other countries ($p < 0.01$), whereas such patients in Italy were significantly fewer [18].

Visual prognosis of patients with ocular BD was extremely poor before the 1970s but has been gradually improving. In a report published in 1970 from Turkey, most ocular BD patients went blind (no light perception) within 5 years after onset [41]. Similarly, in a report in 1979 from Japan, a final best-corrected visual acuity (BCVA) of less than 0.1, indicating loss of useful vision, was seen in 83 % of the patients [7]. However, the ratio of final BCVA of 0.1 or less ranges from 21 to 34 % in recent publications from Japan [37, 42] and 25 % in Turkey [17] and 24 % in the United States [7]. In an international survey of ocular BD, 23 % of the patients had visual acuity of 0.1 or less at the final visit [18]. Also, several recent reports have demonstrated milder disease and improvement in visual prognosis in recent cases with ocular BD as compared to earlier cases [17, 38, 42, 43]. One of the main reasons for improvement in visual prognosis might be better management, such as the early use of immunosuppressive drugs (azathioprine, cyclosporine, etc.) [44] and biologics (infliximab, an anti-TNF-α monoclonal antibody) [35].

4.6 Evaluation of Disease Activity

Since recurrent episodic intraocular inflammation is characteristic in ocular BD, evaluations of disease activity and the efficacy of drugs for ocular disease related to BD are primarily based on frequency of ocular attacks [45–50]. BCVA is also a good index of disease burden, especially in long-term follow-up cases, and generally used for evaluation of ocular BD [38, 46–48, 51]. However, it is not useful for patients who have already lost their vision. As for other secondary endpoints, location of inflammation site (posterior uveitis and panuveitis more severe than anterior uveitis) [12, 50], presence or absence of severe ocular inflammatory signs (hypopyon, involvement of inflammation of retina, macula, or optic disc) [50], and physician impression of the severity of each ocular attack (mild, moderate, severe) [46, 50] are generally used. As for evaluation of the severity of each ocular attack, semiquantitative evaluations based on the numbers of cells in the anterior chamber (0, 0.5+, 1+,2+, 3+, 4+) [52], a vitreous haze chart [53], and with a laser flare meter [54] have been proposed and are generally used.

We recently developed a novel scoring system for uveitis due to BD, termed the Behçet's disease ocular attack score 24 (BOS24) [55]. The BOS24 is used to indicate the severity of each ocular attack. It consists of a total 24 points maximum summarized from 6 parameters of ocular inflammation symptoms, including anterior chamber cells (4 points), vitreous opacity (4 points), peripheral fundus lesions (8 points), posterior pole lesions (4 points), subfoveal lesions (2 points), and optic disc lesions (2 points). As a total sum of BOS24 for each attack in both eyes during a 6-month period, BOS24-6M presents disease activity for the patient during that period of time. This scoring system may be a useful tool for precise evaluation of disease activities in ocular BD.

Meanwhile, a systemic evaluation method has been established. The Behçet's Disease Current Activity Form (BDCAF), one of the most popular methods to measure the activity of BD, uses a 5-point scale (0–4) to classify clinical features (oral ulcers, genital ulcers, ocular lesions, skin lesions, etc.) by doctors during the 4 weeks prior to the day of assessment [56, 57]. However, the definition of each point in that scale is obscure, especially regarding ocular disease activity.

4.7 Therapy

Visual prognosis in patients with ocular BD is poor without appropriate treatment; thus, ophthalmologists have a heavy responsibility when choosing treatments to control intraocular inflammation. BCVA is often a major factor to evaluate whether therapy is a success or should be altered or stopped. The main objectives and strategies of treatment for ocular BD include prompt attenuation of severity of ocular inflammation in the exacerbation phase (acute-phase treatment) and prevention of subsequent ocular inflammatory attacks and reduction of frequency of ocular attacks in the convalescent phase (remission-phase treatment).

Treatment strategies for prevention of ocular attacks vary among countries. In Japan, the primary treatment approach is the use of colchicine and/or cyclosporine [33, 42, 45, 49, 58, 59]. Briefly, 0.5–1.5 mg/day of colchicine is used as the first choice to manage repeated ocular inflammation that does not respond to topical corticosteroids. Cyclosporine usage is initiated at a dose of 5 mg/kg/day in patients who are not responsive to colchicine. Systemic corticosteroids and other immunosuppressant drugs are used solely for cases of very severe ocular disease or neuro-psychiatric/intestinal/vascular BD [42, 58, 59]. However, current approaches have gradually adopted the use of new biological agents such as infliximab in severe cases [49, 50, 60]. On the other hand, the European League against Rheumatism (EULAR) recommendations for management of Behçet's syndrome (BS) were only recently established [61]. Nine recommendations were agreed between the group members, with the following 2 proposed for ocular involvement: (1) any patient with BS and inflammatory eye disease affecting the posterior segment should be on a treatment regime, including azathioprine and systemic corticosteroids, and (2) if the patient has severe eye disease, defined as >2 lines of drop in visual acuity on a 10/10 scale and/or retinal disease (retinal vasculitis or macular involvement), it is recommended that either cyclosporine A or infliximab be used in combination with azathioprine and corticosteroids; alternatively, interferon (IFN)-α with or without corticosteroids could be used instead of that regimen.

4.7.1 *Acute-Phase Treatment*

4.7.1.1 Anterior Ocular Attacks

Patients with isolated anterior uveitis are usually treated with a strong topical corticosteroid (i.e., 0.1 % dexamethasone or betamethasone) and cycloplegic eyedrops. In mild anterior uveitis cases, topical corticosteroids are administrated 4–6 times a day, while in severe cases, those should be used very frequently (every hour) and gradually tapered to 6–12 times daily. In patients with iridocyclitis with hypopyon, a subconjunctival corticosteroid injection should be added. Usually, 1.2–2.0 mg of dexamethasone phosphate solution (Decadron®) is subconjunctivally injected and sometimes repeatedly administrated until a reduction of intraocular inflammation is observed. After several days, the frequency of topical corticosteroid is reduced to 3 or 4 times a day and further reduced according to the decline of anterior chamber inflammation. After 2 or 3 months, topical therapy can be discontinued or switched to a weak topical corticosteroid (0.1 % fluorometholone) or nonsteroidal anti-inflammatory drugs (NSAIDs), such as indomethacin and diclofenac, if cells in the anterior chamber are diminished. Topical cycloplegic agents (i.e., tropicamide-phenylephrine hydrochloride eyedrops) are started at 1–8 times per day, according to the strength of anterior chamber inflammation. When fresh posterior synechia of the iris is observed, frequent administration of a topical cycloplegic agent is recommended for synechiolysis. The frequency of topical cycloplegic agent use is also gradually reduced according to the reduction of anterior chamber inflammation.

4.7.1.2 Posterior Ocular Attacks

As local therapy for an acute ocular attack involving posterior uveitis and/or CME, a posterior sub-Tenon's membrane injection (dexamethasone, 2 mg/0.5 ml) is generally used. This injection is sometimes performed several times to reduce severe tissue damage and retinal edema due to severe ocular attack, which is related to poor visual prognosis. When a physician hopes to continue the effects of the injection for more than 1 month, a depot corticosteroid agent (triamcinolone acetonide or methylprednisolone acetate) should be injected into the posterior sub-Tenon's membrane space, which will cause the effectiveness to continue for 2 or 3 months. Nevertheless, it is necessary to exercise caution against ocular perforation and intraocular pressure elevation.

Topical corticosteroid and cycloplegic agents are also administrated according to the strength of anterior chamber inflammation. However, topical corticosteroids may not reach the required concentration in the posterior segment of the eyes, because penetration of these drugs is poor. On the other hand, sub-Tenon's membrane injection of a corticosteroid agent is considered to penetrate the sclera better than topical corticosteroids.

When an ocular attack of posterior segment inflammation is severe, short-term oral corticosteroid or that by intravenous infusion might be useful to reduce inflammation quickly and rescue the retina and/or optic nerve from tissue damage.

For example, a 3-day intravenous infusion of dexamethasone sodium phosphate (8 mg) can be administrated followed by 30–40 mg of oral prednisolone for 7 days.

4.7.2 *Remission-Phase Treatment*

For patients who repeatedly suffer ocular attacks, systemic treatment is required to prevent subsequent ocular attacks. However, the recommended systemic treatment varies somewhat among countries. Colchicine is the first-line drug used in Japan and may be effective in about 60 % of affected patients [45]. Even when they do not show sufficient effects to suppress ocular inflammation, cyclosporine, oral corticosteroid, azathioprine, and infliximab are considered for administration. However, cyclosporine is not necessarily effective in all patients and has a high incidence of adverse side effects, such as impairment of renal function, central nervous system (CNS) symptoms, and/or liver dysfunction. Therefore, early introduction of infliximab should be considered in severe cases, especially those with threatened sight [62]. Severe cases are considered to be those (1) with a higher frequency of posterior/panuveitis-type ocular attacks, (2) with ocular attacks in the posterior pole, and (3) close to blindness due to advanced visual dysfunction caused by previous inflammation. In European countries, the EULAR recommendations for management of BS [61] are widely accepted and used for remission-phase treatment.

4.7.2.1 Colchicine

Colchicine is an anti-inflammatory plant alkaloid that suppresses neutrophil chemotaxis by inhibiting microtubular function. Administration at 1 mg/day is reported to be effective for suppressing the frequency and/or severity of ocular inflammatory attacks in 60 % of ocular BD patients [45, 63, 64] and is used as a first-line drug for BD treatment in Japan. However, it is not utilized worldwide, likely because its efficacy is questionable, especially for severe posterior uveitis. Moreover, no positive findings in a randomized clinical trial have been presented. In a double-masked open trial, the effect of colchicine was inferior to that of cyclosporine [46]. Thus, colchicine is mainly used in patients with mild to moderately severe ocular disease or treatment for mucocutaneous lesions. Diarrhea and hepatotoxicity are common adverse side effects, while it can rarely induce myopathy and teratogenesis. It is necessary for both men and women to avoid conception/pregnancy during administration.

4.7.2.2 Cyclosporine

Cyclosporine is a product of fungi and an immunosuppressant that selectively inhibits the activation and recruitment of T cells by suppressing intracellular calcineurin. Randomized controlled and masked trials have been performed, which demonstrated that cyclosporine was significantly effective as compared with conventional therapy (azathioprine and/or corticosteroid) [65] and colchicine [46]. With 5–10 mg/kg/day of cyclosporine, the frequency and severity of ocular inflammatory attacks decreased, and visual acuity was significantly improved [46, 65–67]. Based on those results, cyclosporine is widely used for ocular BD, especially in severe cases. However, because higher doses (5–10 mg/kg/day) have frequently induced renal dysfunction [68], a lower dose (5 mg/kg/day or less) is recommended and the blood level should be maintained from 50 to 150 ng/ml. Moreover, a microemulsion pre-concentrate (MEPC) formulation of cyclosporine (Neoral®) was developed to improve intestinal absorption and stabilize fluctuations in blood levels [69]. Other adverse side effects are hirsutism, hepatotoxicity, gastrointestinal disturbances, hypertension, hyperglycemia, and gingival hyperplasia. Especially, attention should be given to neuro-BD-like central nervous system involvement, because the use of cyclosporine may increase that risk [70].

4.7.2.3 Azathioprine

Azathioprine is a mercaptopurine derivate that inhibits an enzyme for purine ring synthesis that is necessary for DNA replication. Thus, it most strongly affects proliferating cells, such as T cells and B cells of the immune system. Oral azathioprine (2.5 mg/kg/day) alone or combination with other immunosuppressants significantly reduced the frequency and severity of ocular disease in a large randomized placebo-controlled trial [71]. Other studies have also demonstrated that azathioprine as monotherapy or in combination with a corticosteroid was effective for controlling retinal vasculitis, as both suppressed involvement of the posterior segment of the eye and improved long-term visual prognoses [72, 73]. Azathioprine is widely used for BD treatment in many countries, though rarely in Japan, especially for ocular disease. Its adverse side effects are hepatotoxicity, gastrointestinal disturbances, and bone marrow suppression.

4.7.2.4 Corticosteroids

Corticosteroids produce a broad nonselective suppression of the immune system by inhibition of the cyclooxygenase and lipoxygenase pathways. They also reduce production of prostaglandins, leukotrienes, and thromboxane in neutrophils and decrease lymphocyte migration and chemotaxis, the number of circulating monocytes, macrophage activity, and the levels of complement and interleukins.

Topical and systemic corticosteroids are commonly used as anti-inflammatory agents for treatment of the vast majority of BD manifestations. However, case–control studies are lacking and the long-term use of a systemic corticosteroid is limited because of potential adverse side effects such as hyperglycemia, osteoporosis, anxiety, and insomnia, which requires alternative use of other immunosuppressive drugs.

A topical corticosteroid is primarily used for ocular inflammatory attacks, though its frequency should be gradually reduced according to the decline in anterior chamber inflammation. Topical therapy is usually discontinued or switched to a weak topical corticosteroid or topical NSAID after a few months.

There is controversy regarding the use of systemic corticosteroids for ocular BD. Single-drug treatment (monotherapy) was routinely performed from the 1950s to 1970s in Japan, though efficacy reports are contradictory [7]. A retrospective study of 414 patients who underwent long-term follow-up examinations clearly indicated that the use of systemic corticosteroids results in poor visual prognosis by induction of ocular attacks with tapering of the drug [74], which was confirmed by others [75, 76]. Thus, systemic corticosteroid monotherapy is discouraged in Japan [7]. However, it was reevaluated in the 1990s, which showed that ocular inflammation can be effectively controlled without induction of ocular attacks in cases treated with low-dose continuous use of oral corticosteroids or combined with other immunosuppressants [77].

Systemic corticosteroid administration is generally accepted in other countries. According to the medical care guidelines for Behçet's disease of EULAR, a prednisolone–azathioprine combination regimen is routinely given as systemic treatment [61]. However, the long-term use of corticosteroid monotherapy might be also avoided in Turkey, because studies there showed that a reduction in dosage can induce ocular attacks with eventual retinal thrombosis and it does not improve visual prognosis [17, 78]. Thus, an oral corticosteroid is usually used with other immunosuppressive drugs and that regimen is thought to have a positive effect on the course of disease by many investigators [77, 79]. However, the long-term use of oral corticosteroids does not avoid adverse side effects, such as secondary cataract formation, elevation of intraocular pressure, hypertension, hyperglycemia, hyperlipidemia, weight gain, Cushing syndrome, gastrointestinal ulcers, osteoporosis, mental status change, and growth retardation in children.

4.7.2.5 Interferon-α-2a

Interferon-α shows immunomodulatory activities such as activation of T cells and natural killer cells and may be helpful for elimination of foreign antigens [80, 81]. Subcutaneous administration of recombinant human interferon-α-2a is often adopted for treatment of refractory BD in Germany, Turkey, and other countries, though it seems to be a suspicious therapeutic strategy [48]. Interferon-α-2a has shown encouraging results for treatment of ocular BD alone or when combined with a corticosteroid and/or immunosuppressants, as those reduced the frequency and severity of ocular attacks [48, 82–84] and improved visual acuity, even in long-term observations averaging 70.6 months [48]. In a clinical trial of 50 cases, 46 (92 %) indicated high efficacy and 20 (40 %) showed remission without the need for further treatments [83]. However, a high incidence of adverse side effects has been noted, including fever, joint pain, and red flares at the injection site in nearly all cases, while 40 % reported leukocytopenia and 24 % eventually suffered from hair loss/alopecia.

4.7.2.6 Chlorambucil

Chlorambucil is a slow-acting alkylating agent that interferes with DNA replication and causes suppression of T- and B-cell function. It is used in BD cases with CNS involvement and severe ocular disease, usually combined with an oral corticosteroid. Although it may improve long-term visual prognosis [85–88], it can also cause severe adverse side effects, especially bone marrow suppression. Thus, usage is limited, especially in severe cases.

4.7.2.7 Anti-TNF-α Biological Agents

TNF-α, a predominant pre-inflammatory cytokine that is produced chiefly by activated macrophages, CD4+ T lymphocytes, and natural killer cells, induces an active phase of inflammatory reaction. It is also a potent chemoattractant for neutrophils and promotes the expression of adhesion molecules on endothelial cells, helping migration of neutrophils. With macrophages, it stimulates phagocytosis and production of interleukin-1 and prostaglandin E2. In BD, production of TNF-α in intraocular T-cell clones and peripheral monocytes was found to be more active in patients with BD accompanied by uveoretinitis than in healthy controls [89]. Furthermore, the ratio of TNF-α-producing cells among peripheral blood mononuclear cells is particularly high in patients with active disease as compared with inactive patients and healthy individuals [90]. These results indicate that TNF-α plays a pivotal role in BD.

Biological agents are drugs that are produced using biotechnology methods. Since they target a single cytokine, there are potential benefits associated with a specific action. Presently, there are 5 biological agents against TNF-α available, a chimeric monoclonal antibody (infliximab), humanized monoclonal antibodies (adalimumab, golimumab), a soluble TNF receptor (etanercept) and a humanised pagylated antibody fragment (certolizumab pegol).

Infliximab is an anti-TNF-α chimeric monoclonal antibody agent used worldwide for treatment of rheumatoid arthritis (RA), Crohn's disease, ulcerative colitis, ankylosing spondylitis, psoriasis, and BD. This agent has a highly suppressive effect on ocular inflammatory attacks as compared to conventional therapy with colchicine and cyclosporine [49] and was approved for refractory uveoretinitis due to BD in Japan in 2007. Other studies have confirmed that patients receiving infliximab therapy showed a significant decrease in frequency of inflammation attacks, improved visual acuity, and reduced ocular complications as compared to those receiving conventional therapy [50, 60, 91–93]. In a control study, the number of relapses was significantly less in the infliximab treatment group than the conventional therapy group that included cyclosporine, azathioprine, and an oral corticosteroid [60, 92]. Moreover, clinical studies of infliximab for BD have shown it to be rapidly effective not only for symptoms of ocular BD [49, 50, 60, 91–93, 115] but also other systemic symptoms, such as oral aphthous ulcers [49, 94], genital ulcers

[95–97], skin lesions [49], arthritis [97], gastrointestinal lesion [97, 98], and CNS involvement [97, 99, 100].

As treatment for BD, 5 mg/kg of infliximab is administered by intravenous infusion and subsequent administrations are performed at 2 and 6 weeks, then every 8 weeks thereafter. Although administration of infliximab strongly suppresses intraocular inflammation, withdrawal of treatment may cause recurrence of ocular attacks [101]. One of the reasons may be that the maintenance of the serum infliximab level is important for suppression of acute uveitis attacks [102].

The main adverse side effects of infliximab treatment are fever, headache, skin rash, hepatotoxicity, and rhinopharyngitis. On the other hand, rare but important adverse side effects include opportunistic infection, reactivation of tuberculosis, infusion reactions during administration, and delayed hypersensitivity to the drug. Moreover, infliximab is contraindicated for active tuberculosis, hepatitis-B virus carriers, nontuberculous mycobacterium, severe congestive cardiac failure, malignant tumors, and demyelination disorders such as multiple sclerosis.

4.7.2.8 Other Treatment Procedures

Granulocyte adsorption therapy (Adacolumn®) employs the passage of venous blood through a column with cellulose beads before returning the blood to the venous system via an extracorporeal circuit, where granulocytes (mainly neutrophils) and monocytes are selectively removed. This therapy is approved in Japan as therapy for ulcerative colitis and Crohn's disease, and with it, the mean frequency of ocular attacks in ocular BD patients has been significantly reduced [103]. Although it lacks dramatic effects, the advantage of this therapy is the absence of severe side effects.

Triamcinolone acetonide (Kenacort-A®) is a slow-release corticosteroid suspension approved for intra-articular injection in patients with rheumatoid arthritis. An intravitreal injection (4 mg) may effectively suppress intraocular inflammation in ocular BD for up to several months, and repeated intravitreous injections completely prevented the recurrence of uveitis in 8 of 9 eyes (89 %) [104]. However, progressive cataracts and increased intraocular pressure are frequently observed. Furthermore, caution is also necessary in regard to possible onset of infectious endophthalmitis. A sub-Tenon's injection of triamcinolone acetonide (20–40 mg) may also be effective for controlling uveitis, along with a lower frequency of adverse side effects [105].

A fluocinolone acetonide intravitreal implant (Retisert®) is designed to deliver therapeutic levels of the drug in the eye over approximately 30 months. It has been approved for chronic noninfectious uveitis affecting the posterior segment of the eye by the FDA of the United States and is expected to provide a suppressive effect for recurrence of uveitis [106]. However, increased frequency of progressive cataracts and intraocular pressure appear inevitable.

4.7.3 *Treatments for Complications*

4.7.3.1 Complicated Cataracts

Complicated cataracts are a frequent complication in patients with ocular BD, especially in cases with strong recurrent ocular attacks. Because ocular inflammation is sometimes induced after surgery, cataract surgery should be performed in cases in which ocular inflammation has not been observed for a period of more than 6 months [106]. Surgical outcome in regard to visual acuity is favorable in most cases [107–109]. In patients with frequent recurrence of uveitis, surgical intervention may be an option 2–4 weeks after an infusion of infliximab [110].

4.7.3.2 Secondary Glaucoma

The mechanism of intraocular pressure elevation in uveitis is due to various etiological factors, such as clogging of inflammatory cells in the trabecular meshwork, overproduction of aqueous humor, corticosteroid treatment, angle occlusion induced by peripheral anterior synechia of the iris, and papillary block [111]. If intraocular pressure could not be controlled with topical or oral antiglaucoma agents, a trabeculectomy or trabeculotomy should be performed after the control of intraocular inflammation. Although there are only a few reports of the efficacy of a trabeculectomy for secondary glaucoma due to ocular BD [112, 113], it might be comparable or slightly worse than that for primary open-angle glaucoma. On the other hand, there are no reports showing the efficacy of a trabeculotomy against secondary glaucoma due to ocular BD; thus, it might be favorable in cases in which intraocular inflammation is well controlled and are suspected to be steroid-induced glaucoma [114].

4.7.3.3 Cystoid Macular Edema (CME)

CME occurs in some BD patients. A dose of 20–40 mg of triamcinolone acetonide (Kenacort-A®) as a sub-Tenon's injection was reported to be effective in 82 % cases with CME due to uveitis and the efficacy may continue for about 3 months [105]. However, it is necessary to exercise caution for adverse side effects such as progression of cataracts, intraocular pressure elevation, blepharoptosis, and ocular perforation.

4.7.3.4 Vitrectomy for Vitreoretinal Complications

It may be necessary to perform a vitrectomy in cases with persistent vitreous hemorrhage, epiretinal membrane, macular hole, or retinal detachment. However, similar to cataract surgery, ocular inflammation may be induced after surgery. Therefore, a vitrectomy is preferred in cases in which an ocular inflammatory attack has not been observed for a period of more than 6 months.

4.8 Summary

Ocular disease associated with BD is one of the most serious problems encountered by affected patients, and the responsibility of the attending ophthalmologist is heavy. Despite therapeutic intervention, about one quarter still lose useful vision, as shown in a recent international survey of ocular BD conducted in 2006 [18]. Actually, visual loss from a severe ocular attack involving the posterior segment of the eye usually occurs suddenly and its prediction is impossible. Thus, the ophthalmologist in charge must adequately evaluate the activity of ocular disease and administer proper medication to prevent the next ocular attack. Earlier therapy may lead to a better prognosis. Notably, the first 2 years after diagnosis of BD is the most critical period for ocular involvement [33, 34]. The goal of treatment of ocular BD is to reduce the frequency and severity of ocular attacks and maintain vision. Fortunately, visual prognosis in recent cases has shown dramatic improvement, especially with introduction of anti-TNF-α biological agents. In light of available biological therapeutics and further development of novel therapeutics, ophthalmologists may soon be able to pursue the goal of complete remission of ocular inflammation and no visual impairment in ocular BD patients.

References

1. Al-Aboosi MM, et al. Behçet's disease: clinical study of Jordanian patients. Int J Dermatol. 1996;35:623–5.
2. Hamdan A, et al. Behçet's disease in Lebanon: clinical profile, severity and two-decade comparison. Clin Rheumatol. 2006;25:364–7.
3. Krause I, et al. Behçet's disease in Israel: the influence of ethnic origin on disease expression and severity. J Rheumatol. 2001;28:1033–6.
4. Kural-Seyahi E, et al. The long-term mortality and morbidity of Behçet syndrome: a 2-decade outcome survey of 387 patients followed at a dedicated center. Medicine (Baltimore). 2003;82:60–76.
5. Mousa AR, et al. Behçet's disease in Kuwait, Arabia. A report of 29 cases and a review. Scand J Rheumatol. 1986;15:310–32.
6. Inaba H. A research report of a National Immunological Survey and an estimate of the number of BD patients (Overcoming intractable disease research project) supported by Scientific Research Grant in aid from the Ministry of Health, Labor, and Welfare. An investigation & research study 2005: an overview and collaborative study report; 2005. p. 89–90. (in Japanese)
7. Mishima S, et al. The eighth Frederick H. Verhoeff Lecture. presented by Saiichi Mishima, MD Behçet's disease in Japan: ophthalmologic aspects. Trans Am Ophthalmol Soc. 1979;77:225–79.
8. Ohguro N, et al. The 2009 prospective multi-center epidemiologic survey of uveitis in Japan. Jpn J Ophthalmol. 2012;56(5):432–5.

9. Soheilian M, et al. Patterns of uveitis in a tertiary eye care center in Iran. Ocul Immunol Inflamm. 2004;12:297–310.
10. Sittivarakul W, et al. Pattern of uveitis in university-based referral center in southern Thailand. Ocul Immunol Inflamm. 2013;21:53–60.
11. Islam SM, et al. Causes of uveitis at The Eye Center in Saudi Arabia: a retrospective review. Ophthalmic Epidemiol. 2002;9:239–49.
12. Mercanti A, et al. Epidemiology of endogenous uveitis in north-eastern Italy. Analysis of 655 new cases. Acta Ophthalmol Scand. 2001;79:64–8.
13. Tran VT, et al. Epidemiology of uveitis in Switzerland. Ocul Immunol Inflamm. 1994;2:169–76.
14. McCannel CA, et al. Causes of uveitis in the general practice of ophthalmology. Am J Ophthalmol. 1996;121:35–46.
15. Biswas J, et al. Pattern of uveitis in a referral uveitis clinic in India. Int Ophthalmol. 1996;20:223–8.
16. Özen S. Vasculopathy, Behçet's syndrome, and familial Mediterranean fever. Curr Opin Rheumatol. 1999;11:393–8.
17. Tugal-Tutkun I, et al. Uveitis in Behçet's disease: an analysis of 880 patients. Am J Ophthalmol. 2004;138:373–80.
18. Kitaichi N, et al. Ocular features of Behcet's disease: an international collaborative study. Br J Ophthalmol. 2007;91(12):1579–82.
19. Nussenblatt RB. Uveitis in Behçet's disease. Int Rev Immunol. 1997;14:67–79.
20. Sakamoto M, et al. Prognostic factors of vision in patients with Behçet's disease. Ophthalmology. 1995;102:317–21.
21. Mocan MC, et al. Keratic precipitate morphology in uveitic syndromes including Behçet's disease as evaluated with in vivo confocal microscopy. Eye. 2009;23(5):1221–7.
22. Benezra D, et al. Treatment and visual prognosis in Behçet's disease. Br J Ophthalmol. 1986;70:589–92.
23. Yurdakul S, et al. The prevalence of Behçet's syndrome in a rural area in northern Turkey. J Rheumatol. 1988;15:820–2.
24. Atmaca LS. Fundus changes associated with Behçet's disease. Graefes Arch Clin Exp Ophthalmol. 1989;227(4):340–4.
25. Yu HG, et al. Fluorescein angiography and visual acuity in active uveitis with Behçet disease. Ocul Immunol Inflamm. 2009;17(1):41–6.
26. Ozdal PC, et al. Posterior segment involvement in ocular Behçet's disease. Eur J Ophthalmol. 2002;12(5):424–31.
27. Keino H, et al. Decreased ocular inflammatory attacks and background retinal and disc vascular leakage in patients with Behcet's disease on infliximab therapy. Br J Ophthalmol. 2011;95(9):1245–50.
28. Nussenblatt RB. Behçet's disease. In: Nussenblatt RB, Whitcup SM, editors. Uveitis: fundamental and practice. Philadelphia: Mosby; 2010. p. 332–54.
29. Takahashi T, et al. A clinical evaluation of uveitis-associated secondary glaucoma. Jpn J Ophthalmol. 2002;46(5):556–62.
30. Elgin U, et al. Incidence of secondary glaucoma in Behçet disease. J Glaucoma. 2004;13:441–4.
31. Al-Dhibi H, et al. Macular hole in Behçet's disease. Indian J Ophthalmol. 2011;59(5):359–62.
32. Tugal-Tutkun I, et al. Neovascularization of the optic disc in Behçet's disease. Jpn J Ophthalmol. 2006;50(3):256–65.
33. Kaburaki T, et al. Best-corrected visual acuity and frequency of ocular attacks during the initial 10 years in patients with Behçet's disease. Graefes Arch Clin Exp Ophthalmol. 2010;248(5):709–14.
34. Evereklioglu C. Current concepts in the etiology and treatment of Behçet disease. Surv Ophthalmol. 2005;50(4):297–350.

35. Taylor SR, et al. Behçet disease: visual prognosis and factors influencing the development of visual loss. Am J Ophthalmol. 2011;152(6):1059–66.
36. Demiroğlu H, et al. Risk factor assessment and prognosis of eye involvement in Behcet's disease in Turkey. Ophthalmology. 1997;104(4):701–5.
37. Takeuchi M, et al. Risk and prognostic factors of poor visual outcome in Behcet's disease with ocular involvement. Graefes Arch Clin Exp Ophthalmol. 2005;243(11):1147–52.
38. Kaçmaz RO, et al. Ocular inflammation in Behçet disease: incidence of ocular complications and of loss of visual acuity. Am J Ophthalmol. 2008;146(6):828–36.
39. Cho YJ, et al. Visual prognosis and risk factors for Korean patients with behcet uveitis. Ophthalmologica. 2008;222(5):344–50.
40. Kaburaki T, et al. Genetic association of HLA-A*2601 with ocular Behçet's disease in Japanese patients. Clin Exp Rheumatol. 2010;28(4 Suppl 60):S39–44.
41. Mamo JG. The rate of visual loss in Behçet's disease. Arch Ophthalmol. 1970;84(4):451–2.
42. Yoshida A, et al. Comparison of patients with Behçet's disease in the 1980s and 1990s. Ophthalmology. 2004;111(4):810–15.
43. Cingu AK, et al. Comparison of presenting features and three-year disease course in Turkish patients with Behçet uveitis who presented in the early 1990s and the early 2000s. Ocul Immunol Inflamm. 2012;20(6):423–8.
44. Ozyazgan Y, et al. Eye disease in Behçet's syndrome. In: Yazuci Y, Yazuci H, editors. Behçet's syndrome. New York: Springer; 2010. p. 73–94.
45. Mizushima Y, et al. Colchicine in Behçet's disease. Lancet. 1977;2(8046):1037.
46. Masuda K, et al. Double-masked trial of cyclosporin versus colchicine and long-term open study of cyclosporin in Behçet's disease. Lancet. 1989;1(8647):1093–6.
47. Ozyazgan Y, et al. Low dose cyclosporin A versus pulsed cyclophosphamide in Behçet's syndrome: a single masked trial. Br J Ophthalmol. 1992;76(4):241–3.
48. Gueudry J, et al. Long-term efficacy and safety of low-dose interferon alpha2a therapy in severe uveitis associated with Behçet disease. Am J Ophthalmol. 2008;146(6):837–44.
49. Ohno S, et al. Efficacy, safety, and pharmacokinetics of multiple administration of infliximab in Behçet's disease with refractory uveoretinitis. J Rheumatol. 2004;31:1362–8.
50. Okada AA, et al. Multicenter study of infliximab for refractory uveoretinitis in Behçet disease. Arch Ophthalmol. 2012;130:592–8.
51. Krause L, et al. Longterm visual prognosis of patients with ocular Adamantiades-Behçet's disease treated with interferon-alpha-2a. J Rheumatol. 2008;35(5):896–903.
52. Jabs DA, Standardization of Uveitis Nomenclature (SUN) Working Group, et al. Standardization of uveitis nomenclature for reporting clinical data. Results of the First International Workshop. Am J Ophthalmol. 2005;140:509–16.
53. Nussenblatt RB, et al. Standardization of vitreal inflammatory activity in intermediate and posterior uveitis. Ophthalmology. 1985;92:467–71.
54. Oshika T, et al. Quantitative assessment of aqueous flare and cells in uveitis. Jpn J Ophthalmol. 1989;33(3):279–87.
55. Kaburaki T, et al. Behçet's disease ocular attack score 24: evaluation of ocular disease activity before and after initiation of infliximab. Jpn J Ophthalmol. 2014;58(2):120–30.
56. Bhakta BB, et al. Behçet's disease: evaluation of a new instrument to measure clinical activity. Rheumatology (Oxford). 1999;38:728–33.
57. Lawton G, et al. The Behcet's disease activity index. Rheumatology (Oxford). 2004;43:73–8.
58. Behçet's Disease Research Committee of Japan. The protocol of treatment and prevention of Behçet's disease. Tokyo: Ministry of Health and Welfare; 1987. p. 22–9 (Japanese).
59. Behçet's Disease Research Committee of Japan. The manual of treatments for Behçet's disease. Tokyo: Ministry of Health and Welfare; 1995. p. 49–51 (Japanese).
60. Yamada Y, et al. Comparison of infliximab versus ciclosporin during the initial 6-month treatment period in Behçet disease. Br J Ophthalmol. 2010;94(3):284–8.

61. Hatemi G, EULAR Expert Committee, et al. EULAR recommendations for the management of Behçet disease. Ann Rheum Dis. 2008;67(12):1656–62.
62. Sfikakis PP, et al. Effect of infliximab on sight-threatening panuveitis in Behçet's disease. Lancet. 2001;358(9278):295–6.
63. Matsumura N, et al. Leucocyte movement and colchicine treatment in Behcet's disease. Lancet. 1975;2:813.
64. Kotter I, et al. Therapy of Behcet's disease. Ger J Ophthalmol. 1996;5:92–7.
65. BenEzra D, et al. Evaluation of conventional therapy versus cyclosporine A in Behçet's syndrome. Transplant Proc. 1988;20(3 Suppl 4):136–43.
66. Caspers-Velu LE, et al. Cyclosporine in Behçet's disease resistant to conventional therapy. Ann Ophthalmol. 1989;21(3):111–18.
67. Kaklamani VG, et al. Treatment of Behçet's disease – an update. Semin Arthritis Rheum. 2001;30(5):299–312.
68. Fukagawa M, et al. Cyclosporine A nephrotoxicity in patients with Behçet's disease. Dev Toxicol Environ Sci. 1986;14:129–33.
69. Fujino Y, et al. Ciclosporin microemulsion preconcentrate treatment of patients with Behçet's disease. Jpn J Ophthalmol. 1999;43(4):318–26.
70. Kotake S, et al. Central nervous system symptoms in patients with Behçet disease receiving cyclosporine therapy. Ophthalmology. 1999;106(3):586–9.
71. Yazici H, et al. A controlled trial of azathioprine in Behçet's syndrome. N Engl J Med. 1990;322(5):281–5.
72. Hamuryudan V, et al. Azathioprine in Behcet's syndrome: effects on long-term prognosis. Arthritis Rheum. 1997;40(4):769–74.
73. Greenwood AJ, et al. The role of azathioprine in the management of retinal vasculitis. Eye (Lond). 1998;12(Pt 5):783–8.
74. Urayama A, et al. Etiology and treatment of Behçet's disease. Acta Soc Ophthalmol Jpn. 1974;78:1304–46 (Japanese).
75. Sugiura S. Some observations on uveitis in Japan, with special reference to Vogt-Koyanagi-Harada and Behçet disease. Acta Soc Ophthalmol Jpn. 1976;80:1285–326 (Japanese).
76. Oniki S. Pathogenesis and treatment of Behçet's disease. Acta Soc Ophthalmol Jpn. 1974;78:1347–78 (Japanese).
77. Whitcup SM, et al. Combined cyclosporine and corticosteroid therapy for sight-threatening uveitis in Behçet's disease. Am J Ophthalmol. 1994;118(1):39–45.
78. Evereklioglu C. Managing the symptoms of Behçet's disease. Expert Opin Pharmacother. 2004;5(2):317–28.
79. Mochizuki M, et al. Behcet's disease. In: Pepose JS, Holland GN, Wilhelmus KR, editors. Ocular inflammation and immunity. St. Louis: Mosby Elsevier; 1996. p. 663–75.
80. O'Duffy JD, et al. Interferon-alpha treatment of Behçet's disease. J Rheumatol. 1998; 25(10):1938–44.
81. Kotter I, et al. The use of interferon-alpha in Behçet's disease – review of the literature and possible mechanisms of action. Adv Exp Med Biol. 2003;528:503–9.
82. Alpsoy E, et al. Interferon-alfa-2α in the treatment of Behçet disease: a randomized placebo-controlled and double-blind study. Arch Dermatol. 2002;138:467–71.
83. Kotter I, et al. Human recombinant interferon alfa-2a for the treatment of Behcet's disease with sight threatening posterior or panuveitis. Br J Ophthalmol. 2003;87:423–31.
84. Tugal-Tutkun I, et al. Results of interferon-alfa therapy in patients with Behçet uveitis. Graefes Arch Clin Exp Ophthalmol. 2006;244:1692–5.
85. O'Duffy JD, et al. Chlorambucil in the treatment of uveitis and meningoencephalitis of Behçet's disease. Am J Med. 1984;76(1):75–84.
86. Elliott JH, et al. Behçet's syndrome: treatment with chlorambucil. Trans Am Ophthalmol Soc. 1984;82:264–81.
87. Zaghetto JM, et al. Chlorambucil and cyclosporine A in Brazilian patients with Behçet's disease uveitis: a retrospective study. Arq Bras Oftalmol. 2010;73(1):40–6.

88. Mudun BA, et al. Short-term chlorambucil for refractory uveitis in Behcet's disease. Ocul Immunol Inflamm. 2001;9(4):219–29.
89. Sagawa K, et al. Production of IL-8 and the other cytokines by T cell clones established from the ocular fluid of patients with Behcet's disease. Ocul Immunol Inflamm. 1995;3:63–71.
90. Misumi M, et al. Cytokine production profile in patients with Behcet's disease treated with infliximab. Cytokine. 2003;24(5):210–18.
91. Tugal-Tutkun I, et al. Efficacy of infliximab in the treatment of uveitis that is resistant to treatment with the combination of azathioprine, cyclosporine, and corticosteroids in Behçet's disease: an open-label trial. Arthritis Rheum. 2005;52(8):2478–84.
92. Tabbara KF, et al. Infliximab effects compared to conventional therapy in the management of retinal vasculitis in Behçet disease. Am J Ophthalmol. 2008;146(6):845–50.
93. Niccoli L, et al. Long-term efficacy of infliximab in refractory posterior uveitis of Behcet's disease: a 24-month follow-up study. Rheumatology (Oxford). 2007;46(7):1161–4.
94. Almoznino G, et al. Infliximab for the treatment of resistant oral ulcers in Behçet's disease: a case report and review of the literature. Clin Exp Rheumatol. 2007;25(4 Suppl 45):S99–102.
95. Haugeberg G, et al. Successful treatment of genital ulcers with infliximab in Behcet's disease. Ann Rheum Dis. 2004;63(6):744–5.
96. Kasugai C, et al. Infliximab treatment of severe genital ulcers associated with Behçet disease. J Am Acad Dermatol. 2010;62(1):162–4.
97. Donghi D, et al. Infliximab for the treatment of refractory Adamantiades-Behçet disease with articular, intestinal, cerebral and ocular involvement. Dermatology. 2010;220(3):282–6.
98. Iwata S, et al. Effects of anti-TNF-alpha antibody infliximab in refractory entero-Behcet's disease. Rheumatology (Oxford). 2009;48(8):1012–13.
99. Abalos-Medina GM, et al. Successful use of infliximab in a patient with neuro-Behçet's disease. Int J Rheum Dis. 2009;12(3):264–6.
100. Pipitone N, et al. Infliximab for the treatment of Neuro-Behçet's disease: a case series and review of the literature. Arthritis Rheum. 2008;59(2):285–90.
101. Adán A, et al. Effects of infliximab in the treatment of refractory posterior uveitis of Behçet's disease after withdrawal of infusions. Int Ophthalmol. 2010;30(5):577–81.
102. Sugita S, et al. Relationship between serum infliximab levels and acute uveitis attacks in patients with Behcet disease. Br J Ophthalmol. 2011;95(4):549–52.
103. Namba K, et al. Granulocytapheresis in patients with refractory ocular Behcet's disease. J Clin Apher. 2006;21:121–8.
104. Ohguro N, et al. Repeated intravitreal triamcinolone injections in Behcet disease that is resistant to conventional therapy: one-year results. Am J Ophthalmol. 2006;141:218–20.
105. Okada AA, et al. Trans-Tenon's retrobulbar triamcinolone infusion for the treatment of uveitis. Br J Ophthalmol. 2003;87(8):968–71.
106. Jaffe GJ, et al. Fluocinolone acetonide implant (Retisert) for noninfectious posterior uveitis: thirty-four-week results of a multicenter randomized clinical study. Ophthalmology. 2006;113:1020–7.
107. Matsuo T, et al. Ocular attacks after phacoemulsification and intraocular lens implantation in patients with Behçet disease. Ophthalmologica. 2001;215(3):179–82.
108. Kadayifçilar S, et al. Cataract surgery in patients with Behçet's disease. J Cataract Refract Surg. 2002;28(2):316–20.
109. Berker N, et al. Phacoemulsification cataract extraction and intraocular lens implantation in patients with Behçet's disease. Ophthalmic Surg Lasers Imaging. 2004;35(3):215–18.
110. Sakai T, et al. Intraocular surgery in patients receiving infliximab therapy for Behçet disease. Jpn J Ophthalmol. 2010;54(4):360–1.
111. Moorthy RS, et al. Glaucoma associated with uveitis. Surv Ophthalmol. 1997; 41(5):361–94.
112. Elgin U, et al. Trabeculectomy with mitomycin C in secondary glaucoma associated with Behçet disease. J Glaucoma. 2007;16(1):68–72.

113. Iwao K, et al. Long-term outcomes and prognostic factors for trabeculectomy with mitomycin C in eyes with uveitic glaucoma: a retrospective cohort study. J Glaucoma. 2014; 23(2):88–94.
114. Iwao K, et al. Success rates of trabeculotomy for steroid-induced glaucoma: a comparative, multicenter, retrospective cohort study. Am J Ophthalmol. 2011;151(6):1047–56.
115. Accorinti M, et al. Infliximab treatment for ocular and extraocular manifestations of Behçet's disease. Jpn J Ophthalmol. 2007;51(3):191–6.

Chapter 5
Vascular Involvement of Behçet's Disease

Mitsuhiro Takeno, Haruko Ideguchi, Akiko Suda, Reikou Kamiyama, and Yoshiaki Ishigatsubo

Abstract Vascular involvement is found in 6.3–51.6 % of the patients with Behçet's disease (BD). It can be serious in some patients, especially in young-aged male patients. The lesions are distributed in the both arterial and venous systems, regardless of the size. Deep vein thrombosis (DVP) is the most characteristic, whereas superficial thrombophlebitis is considered as one of the cutaneous symptoms. DVP is located in any anatomical site, including superior and inferior vena cava, cerebral sinus, hepatic veins, and so on. Arterial lesions typically form aneurysms and occlusion. Peripheral arterial and pulmonary arterial aneurysms often lead to lethal events, whereas the occlusive lesions are negatively associated with remission. Cardiac involvement is also critical, though the incidence is rare. These lesions are illustrated by various imaging modalities such as angiography, CT scan, ultrasonography, MRI, and PET.

Because inflammation is the most important of underlying pathological changes in any type of vascular lesions, corticosteroids and immunosuppressants are used as first-line therapies. Recent reports have suggested that tumor necrosis factor (TNF) inhibitors are promising as an option. Surgical operation is necessary for impending rupture of aneurysm, though the procedures are frequently complicated with post-operative recurrence of aneurysm and occlusions. Endovascular intervention is an alternative with a lower incidence of complications. Use of anticoagulants and anti-platelets is controversial, because clinical efficacy of the agents has not been proven, and they may increase risk of fatal hemoptysis from pulmonary arterial aneurysms which frequently coexists.

M. Takeno, M.D., Ph.D. (✉) • R. Kamiyama, M.D. • Y. Ishigatsubo, M.D., Ph.D.
Department of Internal Medicine and Clinical Immunology, Yokohama City University Graduate School of Medicine, 3-9 Fukuura, Kanazawa-Ku, Yokohama 236-0004, Japan
e-mail: m2takeno@med.yokohama-cu.ac.jp

H. Ideguchi, M.D., Ph.D.
Department of Internal Medicine and Clinical Immunology, National Hospital Organization Yokohama Medical Center, 3-60-2, Harajuku, Totuka-Ku, Yokohama 236-0004, Japan

A. Suda, M.D., Ph.D.
Center for Rheumatic Diseases, Yokohama City University Medical Center, 4-57, Urafune, Minami-Ku, Yokohama 236-0004, Japan

Y. Ishigatsubo (ed.), *Behçet's Disease*,
DOI 10.1007/978-4-431-54487-6_5

Keywords Aneurysm • Deep vein thrombosis • Immunosuppressants • Recurrence • Anticoagulants

5.1 Introduction

Vasculitis is considered as the underlying nature of Behçet's disease (BD) [1]. The concept of vasculo-Behçet disease has been adopted for those cases in which involvement of great vessels dominates the clinical features. It has been controversial whether the vascular involvement should be incorporated into the International Study Group for BD criteria set [2], but it is not included because of the low sensitivity. In the Japanese Diagnostic Criteria for BD, vascular involvement is listed as one of 5 minor symptoms [3]. Moreover, vasculo-BD as well as neuro-BD and intestinal BD are categorized into the special types, in which clinical outcomes and prognosis are unfavorable if therapy is inappropriate [3].

Because of the heterogeneous features, BD vasculitis is classified into variable vessel vasculitis in 2012 Revised International Chapel Hill Consensus Conference Nomenclature of Vasculitides [4]. The disease can affect vessels of any size and type. Small-vessel vasculitis, arteritis, arterial aneurysms, and venous and arterial thromboangiitis and thrombosis may occur [4]. When compared with other types of vasculitis syndromes, venous vascular involvement is the most unique feature of BD. Moreover, pulmonary arterial aneurysm (PAA) and thrombosis are also found in some patients [5–7]. Broad spectrum of lesion distribution causes diverse clinical symptoms, from mild to severe. The most serious form of vascular involvement, such as arterial lesions and pulmonary artery aneurysms, is associated with mortality and morbidity in BD [5–12].

EULAR recommendations for management of BD included two statements for vascular diseases of BD [13]. The statements recommend immunosuppressive therapies for both arterial and venous involvement, whereas use of anticoagulants, antiplatelet, or antifibrinolytic agents are not encouraged [13–15]. Rather, the recommendations referred to avoiding these agents, because of low incidence of pulmonary embolisms and risk of fatal bleeding from coexisting pulmonary aneurysms [7, 12, 16]. Because these statements are based on expert opinions rather than evidence, they have to be validated in different countries and different setting as noted in the EULAR recommendations [13]. Indeed, there are some reports suggesting different opinions [3, 8, 17–19]. Moreover, there is no comment on surgical operation and endovascular interventions, both of which are required in some cases, especially in emergencies.

In this chapter, we focus on the serious form of vascular involvement, so-called vasculo-BD and review the clinical features and the diagnostic procedures and discuss the treatment.

5.2 Epidemiology and Classification of Vascular Involvement in BD

Previous studies from different ethnic groups have reported that the prevalence of vascular involvement varies from 6.3 to 51.6 % in all phenotypes of BD patients (Table 5.1) [3, 8, 11, 16, 20–27]. Differences in the frequency among the reports may be from the ethnic differences, besides study designs including definition of vascular involvement and clinical evaluation techniques. The vascular lesions usually develop as late manifestations of the disease [3, 8, 11, 21, 28]. In our series, vascular lesions developed 2.2±8.4 years after diagnosis of patients [3], but they can appear as the initial manifestations. Young-aged onset and male are identified as independent predispositions to vascular involvement [8, 9, 11, 18, 28, 29].

Venous lesions are more common than arterial lesions as shown by all reported studies except a postmortem analysis (Table 5.1) [3, 8, 11, 16, 20–27]. Calamia

Table 5.1 Frequency of vascular involvement in BD patients

	Country	Year	Total BD patients	Total vasculo-BD patients	Arterial involvement	Venous involvement	Reference
Clinical study							
	Japan	1972	2,031	142 (7 %)	–	–	[20]
	Japan	1991	3,316	298 (9 %)	–	–	[20]
Koç et al.	Turkey	1992	137	27 (19.7 %)	5 (4 %)	22 (16 %)	[21]
al-Dalaan et al.	Saudi Arabia	1994	119	37 (31.1 %)	22 (18 %)	30 (25 %)	[22]
Gürler et al.	Turkey	1997	2,147	222 (10.3 %)	25 (1 %)	197 (9 %)	[23]
Kural-Seyahi et al.	Turkey	2003	387	88 (22.7 %)	21 (5 %)	82 (21 %)	[11]
Tohmé et al.	Lebanon	2003	140	18 (13 %)	6 (4 %)	17 (12 %)	[24]
Düzgün et al.	Turkey	2006	180	71 (39.4 %)	20 (11 %)	68 (38 %)	[25]
Sarica-Kucukoglu et al.	Turkey	2006	2,319	155 (6.7 %)	24 (1 %)	140 (6 %)	[26]
Ideguchi et al.	Japan	2011	412	26 (6.3 %)	8 (2 %)	21 (5 %)	[3]
Saddoum et al.	France, Tunisia	2012	820	315 (38 %)	101 (12 %)	296 (36 %)	[8]
Zhang et al.	China	2013	334	58 (17.4)	26 (8 %)	36 (11 %)	[27]
Autopsy study							
Lakhanpal et al.	Japan	1985	170	74 (43.5 %)	57 (34 %)	17 (10 %)	[16]

Table 5.2 Classification of vascular involvement of Behçet's disease

1. Systemic arterial vasculitis
(a) Aneurysms
(b) Stenosis/occlusions
2. Pulmonary arterial involvement
(a) Aneurysms
(b) Stenosis/occlusions
3. Venous occlusions
(a) Superficial venous thrombosis
(b) Deep vein thrombosis
(c) Vena cava thrombosis
(d) Cerebral venous thrombosis
(e) Budd-Chiari syndrome
(f) Portal vein thrombosis
(g) Right ventricular thrombosis
(h) Pulmonary emboli
4. Varices

et al. proposed the classification of vascular lesions in BD shown in Table 5.2 based on the anatomical sites and the pathology [30]. Of them, superficial thrombophlebitis is categorized as cutaneous symptoms in the Japan BD diagnostic criteria, because the clinical manifestation is not as serious as that in other lesions [3]. However, the presence of superficial thrombophlebitis is considered as a risk factor of future vascular events.

Pulmonary arterial vasculitis is separated from that in the systemic arterial circulation, because of the characteristics of vessels and distinctive presentation. Thrombotic occlusion, stenosis, and aneurysms develop in both systemic and pulmonary circulations. Multiple vascular lesions commonly coexist, indicating that the presence of venous thrombosis, including superficial thrombophlebitis, should be considered as a risk factor of future vascular events [9–11]. Positive or negative association of vascular involvement with extravascular manifestations has been also shown. Patients with vasculo-BD exhibited lower frequency of eye involvement [3, 25], and higher frequency of gastrointestinal involvement [3, 24], compared with the other types of BD patients. Positive pathergy test is also more frequent in vasculo-BD patients than the others, although it might be associated with male predominance rather than clinical phenotypes [3, 21, 31, 32]. In spite of these predispositions, it is not easy to identify high-risk patients who may potentially develop the serious vascular involvement in advance.

5.3 Systemic Arterial Lesions

According to previous large-scale clinical studies examining more than 100 patients, the incidence has been reported from 1 to 18 % and less frequent than venous lesions [3, 8, 11, 16, 20–27]. Arterial involvement, male gender, and frequent clinical flares are independently associated with mortality in BD [9, 11, 33]. Young-aged males and preexisting venous involvement are identified as major predisposing factors for the development of arterial involvement [8–11]. Saadoun et al. showed that up to 80 % of cases affected by the arterial involvement were young men with venous involvement [8]. The reason for male predominance remains uncertain, though implication of estrogen has been suggested in a rat animal model of endotoxin-induced uveitis [34].

5.3.1 Clinical Manifestations

The most prevalent site of arterial involvement is the aorta, followed by pulmonary arteries, femoral, popliteal, and carotid arteries [8, 11, 21, 22, 25, 26, 29, 35]. The lesion can be isolated, but one-third of arterial lesions are multiple [8]. Aneurysms are more frequent than occlusions, though the reverse has been reported [24, 36]. Systemic symptoms such as fever and fatigue and biological inflammatory syndrome, in which CRP and ESR are elevated, are frequently found in the onset of arterial involvement [8].

Aneurysms are caused by vasculitis in the vasa vasorum [16, 37, 38]. Although aneurysms are most commonly found in the abdominal aorta, several reports have shown that thoracic aorta is rarely affected in BD, unlike Takayasu's arteritis [39–41]. On the other hand, acute aortitis or dilatation of the ascending aorta has been shown to cause aortic valve dysfunction which requires surgical operation [42, 43].

Peripheral arterial aneurysms are mostly saccular punched-out pseudoaneurysms with or without thrombosis and are manifested as a painful, hyperemic, pulsating mass. The lesions have the risk of rupture or leakage, but do not cause distal ischemia [37]. Of note, traumatic injuries including arterial puncture, surgery, or angiography often cause arterial lesions, particularly aneurysms [8, 35, 44–48]. The complications are thought to reflect the pathergy phenomenon of BD, suggesting preferential application of noninvasive imaging procedures to prove arterial lesions.

In contrast, abdominal aortic aneurysms are often found in the later stages, because of lack of specific symptoms [37]. On physical examinations, pulsating abdominal mass or audile bruits can be a clue to the diagnosis, though it is sometimes hard to detect the lesions because they may localize posterior regions or be surrounded by the fibrous tissue [37].

Arterial occlusions or stenosis may be asymptomatic or associated with ischemic symptoms, depending on the site of involvement and collateral circulation. Local pain, abdominal pain, fever, loss of pulse, intermittent claudication, skin ulcers, or hemiplegia can appear [29, 47, 48]. Acute myocardial infarction has also been reported [49–54]. Saadoun et al. showed that the occlusive lesions were negatively associated with complete remission [8].

5.3.2 Pathology

In early stages, neutrophils and lymphocytes, predominately CD3+ T cells, intensively infiltrate in the media and adventitia of arterial wall [37, 38]. Vasculitis in the vasa vasorum causes the occlusion and subsequently transmural necrosis, resulting in pseudoaneurysm formation [16, 37, 38]. In chronic stages, the intimal, adventitial, and preadventitial fibrosis is accompanied by the destruction of the media, leading to occlusion in some cases [37]. Unlike Takayasu's arteritis, granulomatous inflammation and marked thickening of the all layers of aorta are not found [41].

5.3.3 *Imaging Diagnosis*

The diagnosis of arterial lesions is made on the basis of imaging modalities. In addition to local assessment, screening of additional lesions in other vessels is recommended, because the vascular lesions can be multiple [8]. Although percutaneous angiography used to be a standard technique to prove arterial lesions, the procedure should be avoided because there is accumulating evidence that arterial puncture increases the risk of the local aneurysm formation [8, 35, 44–48]. Endovascular intervention for therapeutic purposes is exceptional. Instead, intravenous digital subtraction angiography (DSA), contrast-enhanced CT scan angiography including 3 dimensional analysis, MR angiography, and ultrasonography are currently used to illustrate the lesions (Figs. 5.1 and 5.2). Positron emission tomography (PET) and PET-CT scan are promising for the diagnosis and assessment of vasculo-BD, because the imaging modalities are useful for other types of large-vessel vasculitis [3, 55–57].

5.3.4 *Differential Diagnosis*

Because arterial involvement appears as a late complication of the disease, the diagnosis is not hard after establishing BD as the underlying disease. On the other, it is difficult to make the diagnosis when the arterial lesion develops as the initial manifestations or in patients who do not have typical BD manifestations. Large-vessel vasculitis such as Takayasu's arteritis and giant-cell arteritis and middle-size vessel vasculitis such as polyarteritis nodosum should be differentiated. Because coexistence of venous involvement and extravascular manifestations of BD are most helpful, these features should be monitored carefully.

5.4 Venous Lesions

The prevalence of venous involvement is reported from 5 to 38 %, which is higher than arterial involvement in clinical studies form different countries [3, 16, 18, 20–27]. Like other vascular involvement, males are more frequently affected in BD [11, 18, 21, 26, 58, 59]. The venous lesions can be multiple and coexistence of lesions in the arterial and pulmonary systems is also common [5, 7, 10]. The onset of venous involvement is younger than that of arterial involvement [11].

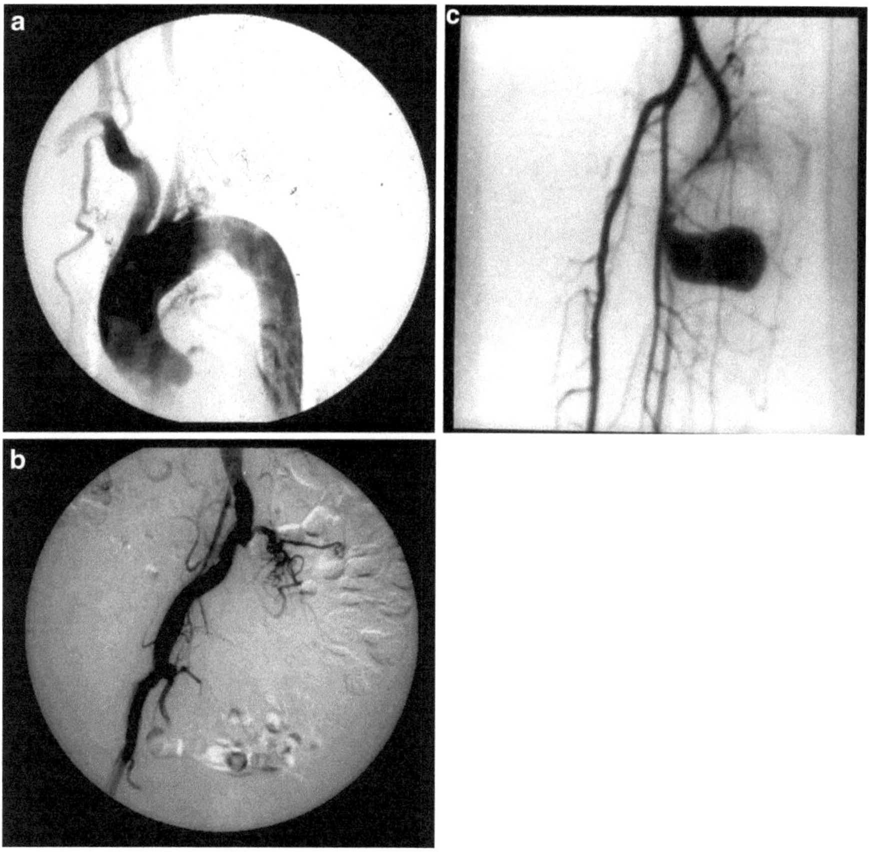

Fig. 5.1 Angiographic findings of arterial lesions. (**a**) Left subclavian artery occlusion (DSA), (**b**) left common iliac artery occlusion (DSA), (**c**) aneurysm in peroneal artery

A study from the UK has reported that BD patients had a 14-fold risk of venous thrombosis compared to controls [60], though the prevalence is different among ethnics. As shown in idiopathic venous thrombosis and those with systemic lupus erythematosus, venous thrombosis in BD patients is more common in Caucasians or African-Americans than in Asian BD patients, suggesting a common genetic susceptibility is involved in thrombogenesis [61, 62]. Although implication of a factor V Leiden mutation [63, 64] and the prothrombin gene mutation [65], both of which are rarely found in Asian populations, have been discussed, contributions of these genetic factors to thrombogenesis in BD are unlikely [66, 67]. No genetic thrombophilic factors have been identified in BD.

Unlike idiopathic venous thrombosis, male predominance is one of the features in BD, suggesting less contribution of sex hormones to thrombogenesis. Rather, inflammation associated vascular damages or endothelial dysfunction may be implicated in thrombogenesis in BD [68–70].

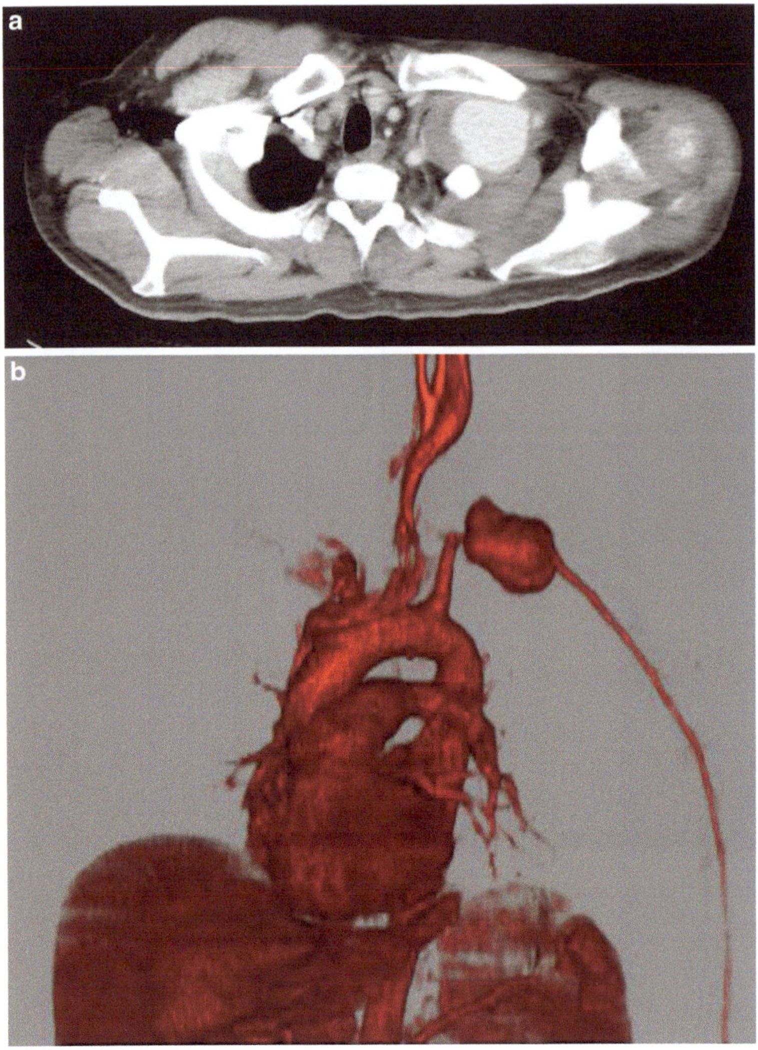

Fig. 5.2 Left subclavian artery aneurysms in contrast CT (**a**) and 3 dimensional CT scan (**b**)

5.4.1 *Clinical Pictures*

Deep vein thrombosis (DVT) occurs more frequently in the legs, especially in popliteal and superficial femoral veins, followed by tributary veins of the calves, common femoral, external iliac, and common iliac veins [3, 18, 26, 36]. The lesions cause local pain, swelling, stasis dermatitis, and skin ulcers.

Venous thrombosis can be distributed in any anatomical site. In superior and inferior vena caval (SVC and IVC) thrombosis, BD should be included in differential diagnosis [56, 71]. SVC thrombosis causes characteristic signs and symptoms of SVC syndrome, in which facial swelling and cyanosis of the face, neck, and upper

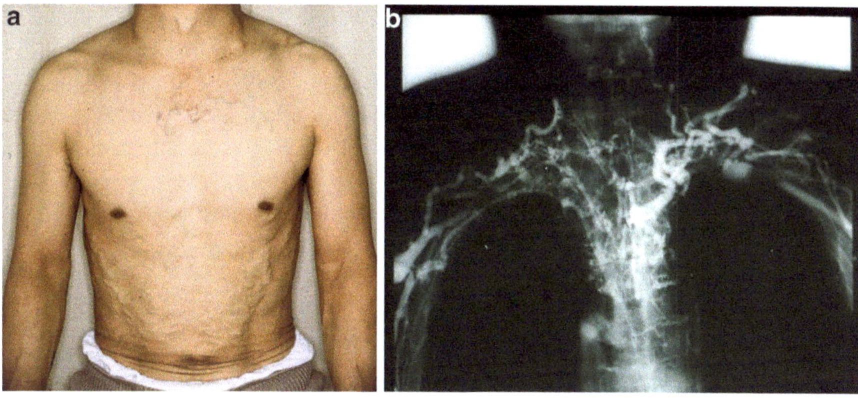

Fig. 5.3 Superior vena cava syndrome. (**a**) Superficial collateral veins, (**b**) venography

limbs with prominent venous collateral circulation, chylothorax, and chylopericardium are found [72–74] (Fig. 5.3). The clinical course of these complications is generally favorable, but can be associated with more serious vascular involvement.

Budd-Chiari syndrome, which is caused by hepatic vein thrombosis, is the most serious venous involvement in BD, though the incidence is rare [8, 18, 75, 76]. A recent study form France identified 4 deaths in 14 patients with Budd-Chiari syndrome of a total of 296 BD patients having venous involvement [18]. Thus, the syndrome in BD patients can be fatal in spite of potent immunosuppressive therapies [18, 77].

Cerebral venous thrombosis (CVT) leads to a neurological manifestation which is categorized into non-parenchymal type of neuro-BD [33, 78–80]. Frequent complication of CVT with other venous involvement may be responsible for significant association between vascular and neurological manifestations [33, 78], though this type of neuro-BD is extremely rare in Japan [20].

5.4.2 Imaging Diagnosis

Contrast-enhanced CT scan, MRA, and ultrasonography are useful for illustrating thrombotic lesions [3].

5.4.3 Differential Diagnosis

Venous thrombosis is caused by various clinical settings including inherited thrombophilia and acquired disorders such as malignancy, heart failure, hematological diseases, and drug-related hypercoagulability. When patients obviously have these clinical setting, it is not hard to differentiate these conditions from BD. On the other hand, when the diagnosis of BD is not established, inherited thrombophilia such as factor V Leiden mutation, prothrombin gene mutations, protein S deficiency, protein C deficiency, and antithrombin deficiency might be considered.

Immune-mediated or inflammatory disorders should be considered as differential diagnosis. Antiphospholipid antibody syndrome (APS) causes thrombotic lesions in both arterial and venous systems like vasculo-BD, though most of the patients are female [81]. Rather, it is important to differentiate inflammatory bowel diseases complicating with venous and arterial thrombosis from BD, especially in east Asian countries where intestinal involvement of BD is prevalent [82], because our cohort study showed significant association between vascular and intestinal lesions [3].

5.5 Pulmonary Arterial Involvement

Pulmonary artery involvement causes PAA, which is one of the most critical complications of BD [5–9, 11, 12], and pulmonary artery thrombosis (PAT) with or without PAA [5–7]. Seyahi et al. retrospectively identified 47 patients with pulmonary artery involvement from about 2,500 patients in Turkey [7, 83–85]. Of them, 34 patients (72 %) presented with PAA, including 8 with associated PAT, whereas the remaining 13 patients had isolated PAT. In addition, pulmonary involvement accompanies additional lung lesions such as nodules, consolidations, and cavity formation in some patients. Lung parenchymal lesions such as organizing pneumonia have been rarely reported [5–7, 10, 12]. Pulmonary artery involvement is prevalent in young-aged males [5–7, 10, 12]. Pulmonary artery involvement develops several years later, after the diagnosis of BD in most of patients, though it may appear as the initial manifestations preceding the other manifestations of BD for several years [7, 86–88].

5.5.1 Clinical Manifestations

Hemoptysis is the most common symptom followed by cough, fever, dyspnea, and pleuritic chest pain [7]. Hemoptysis can be life threatening when PAA is ruptured and is more common in patients with PAA than those with isolated PAT [5–7, 10, 12], though PAT often progresses to PAA, leading to massive bleeding.

Coexistence of other vascular involvement is common [5–7, 10]. Especially, venous thrombosis is found in around 80 % of the patients, whereas the frequency is around 25 % of all BD patients [7]. Vena cava thrombosis, intracardiac thrombosis, and peripheral arterial aneurysms have been complicated. However, embolism is thought to be rare in BD, because the thrombosis is tightly adhered to the endothelium in the diseased veins [68–70].

5.5.2 Pathology

Inflammatory cells, mainly mononuclear cells, infiltrate into the vasa vasorum of the pulmonary arteries, leading to ischemia of the affected arteries and subsequent aneurysm formation [7, 10, 89, 90]. Unlike aneurysms of the peripheral arteries,

PAA is usually a true aneurysm surrounded by dense adventitial fibrosis. Development of bronchiolitis obliterans and organizing pneumonia (BOOP)-like lesions has been reported as rare pulmonary involvement of BD, which is considered to be associated with pulmonary artery lesions [7, 83–85, 89].

5.5.3 *Imaging Diagnosis*

Chest X-ray shows hilar opacities, peripheral nodules or consolidations, and pleural effusions at the onset of pulmonary artery involvement, though no abnormalities are found in some patients, particularly those with isolated PAT, but not with PAA [7, 89–91]. Nodular lesions usually resolve quickly and are considered as BOOP-like lesions, whereas cavities appear persistent [7, 83–85].

Contrast CT illustrates that both the PAA and PAT locate mainly in the descending branches of the pulmonary arteries and mural thrombosis as a common finding [7, 89–91]. PAA are often multiple and bilateral [5–9, 11, 12]. On the other hand, percutaneous transarterial pulmonary angiography is not recommended because of the risk of the local aneurysm formation except when endovascular interventions are indicated [8, 35, 46–48]. Rather, intravenous DAS and MR angiography are useful for showing thrombosed and nonthrombosed pulmonary aneurysms [7, 89–91]. Ventilation-perfusion scintigraphy is helpful for pulmonary artery occlusion [92, 93]. FDG-PET/CT is a promising tool to assess inflammatory activity of pulmonary arteries and parenchymal pulmonary lesions in BD despite limited experience [94, 95]. A recent study has shown that ultrasonography or CT illustrated intracardiac thrombi in one-third of patients with PAA and/or PAT [7]. The imaging modalities are not only useful for making diagnosis but also for monitoring the disease activity, because most of the findings regress or disappear in response to immunosuppressive treatment.

5.5.4 *Differential Diagnosis*

Pulmonary artery involvement generally develops as a late complication of BD and is accompanied by other active signs of BD besides the lung lesions. Therefore, making the diagnosis is not difficult in typical cases. However, hemoptysis, the most frequent symptom, is caused by lung cancer, bronchiectasis, and various infectious diseases including pulmonary tuberculosis and fungal infections. These diseases should be differentiated before initiating or adding intensive therapy. Although imaging modalities are helpful for the differential diagnosis, it is of note that nodular lesions, cavity formation, and even parenchymal opacities are found in pulmonary involvement of BD. Moreover, complications with infections, including reactivation of latent tuberculosis, should be taken into consideration in BD patients receiving potent immunosuppressive therapies [10, 12].

The diagnosis is often difficult especially when the pulmonary lesion appears as the initial manifestation of BD. In such cases, it is impossible to make the diagnosis of BD until other characteristic symptoms appear. Rather, the diagnosis of Hughes-Stovin syndrome is often made in patients presenting PAA and venous thrombosis without extravascular features of BD [86–88]. Interestingly, the lesions show histopathological features similar to those in PAA of BD and respond to immunosuppressive therapies including corticosteroids and cyclophosphamide, azathioprine, and colchicine. Because of the histopathological and clinical similarity, Hughes-Stovin syndrome is likely to be an incomplete form of BD, which requires aggressive therapy for pulmonary lesions.

5.6 Cardiac Involvement

Although cardiac lesions of BD have been reported sporadically as case reports, Geri et al. recently reported a series of 52 consecutive BD patients with cardiac involvement [96]. Cardiac involvement occurs in 1–6 % of BD patients, most often in men, and frequently associated with arterial and venous involvement [96]. Cardiac abnormalities in BD include pericarditis, myocarditis with conducting system findings, endocarditis with valvular regurgitation, intracardiac thrombosis, endomyocardial fibrosis, coronary arteritis, or sinus of Valsalva [16, 40, 96, 97]. Prognosis is significantly poor in BD patients with cardiac lesions than those without the lesions [96]. However, latent lesions may be more common because a postmortem study revealed 16.5 % cardiac involvement in BD [16]. In the study, cardiomegaly was the most common cardiac abnormality, followed by coronary arteritis or thrombosis, endocarditis, pericardial effusion, myocardial fibrosis, and aortic valve disease [16]. Moreover, a clinical study using treadmill exercise test and thallium-201 myocardial perfusion single-photon emission computed tomography has shown that silent myocardial ischemia is found in 19.5 % of BD patients, compared to 2.9 % of age- and sex-matched healthy controls [98], suggesting that latent cardiac involvement of BD is not rare in concordance with the postmortem study.

Pericarditis is the most frequent cardiac feature, accounting for up to 40 % of cardiac involvement [40, 96, 97, 99]. It is typically accompanied by chest pain and fever followed by rapid resolution, but recurrence is common [96]. It can be also asymptomatic [99]. Constrictive pericarditis is rarely reported [100]. Sporadic reports have shown BD can also involve the conduction system, resulting in complete A-V block requiring a permanent pacemaker [101, 102].

Endocardial lesions often cause mitral and aortic valve insufficiency, resulting in valve insufficiency as a serious complication [40, 96, 103, 104]. Valvulitis, aneurysm of the sinus of Valsalva, and aortitis are involved in the process [40, 56, 96]. Aortic regurgitation due to BD usually requires surgical operation, but the postoperative complications are frequent [3, 105–109]. Valve dehiscence after atrial valve replacement and postoperative leakage requiring reoperation are not rare [104–110]. Several studies have suggested that aortic root replacement and postoperative immunosuppressive therapy contribute to improving the therapeutic outcomes of AR in BD patients [109, 110].

Coronary artery lesions, which include stenosis, occlusion, and pseudoaneurysm, are usually proximal, leading to ischemic cardiomyopathy including myocardial infarction [51, 52, 96] and ventricular aneurysm [51, 111, 112]. The clinical outcome is unfavorable. Myocardial infarction can occur in young males, even children having no conventional coronary risk factors [113]. Endomyocardial fibrosis, which is rarely reported, may be a sequelae of vasculitis involving endocardium and/or myocardium and intraventricular thrombosis [40, 96, 114–116]. Surgical resection under immunosuppressive therapies has been shown to be effective.

Intracardiac thrombosis is often reported as a rare and serious complication of BD mainly from the Mediterranean basin and the Middle East. It affects mainly young male patients presenting with fever, dyspnea, and cough [7, 96, 114, 117, 118]. These symptoms can be the initial manifestation of BD in half of the patients. Thrombosis is usually located in the right atrium and ventricle, though the left ventricle can be also involved. In about a half of the patients, PAA and DVT coexist. Histological studies reveal an organizing thrombus containing infiltrating mononuclear cells, suggesting it develops secondary to underlying endocarditis. Indeed, the lesions responded well to immunosuppressive therapies.

5.7 Treatment

Immunosuppressive therapy plays a central role of management of vasculo-BD patients. However, it is controversial whether anticoagulation is beneficial or harmful. Moreover, some patients with arterial involvement such as impending rupture of aneurysms require surgical operation, though postoperative complication and local relapse are very frequent. Endovascular intervention can be an alternative. Accumulating experience has suggested that TNF inhibition is a promising strategy for vasculo-BD.

5.7.1 Immunosuppressive Therapy

In EULAR recommendations, a statement recommends immunosuppressive therapies as follows [13]:

"There is no firm evidence to guide the management of major vessel disease in BD. For the management of acute deep vein thrombosis in BD immunosuppressive agents such as corticosteroids, azathioprine, cyclophosphamide or cyclosporine A are recommended."

This statement is supported by a number of cohort studies and case series [7, 8, 12, 14, 18], though no randomized controlled studies, which may be difficult for vasculo-BD patients, have been shown. Saadoun et al. have shown that use of immunosuppressants such as cyclophosphamide and azathioprine increased by four times the likelihood of complete remission in BD patients with arterial involvement, though half of them underwent a surgical procedure [8].

Because PAA is the leading cause of mortality of BD, early diagnosis and therapy are essential. Yazici H et al. have sequentially reported clinical outcomes of PAA in 1994, 2004, and 2012 in a single institute [7, 10, 12]. In the first report, 12 of 24 patients with PAA (50 %) died after a mean of 9.5+11 months (range 1–36) [12], whereas 6 of 26 patients (23 %), who were diagnosed after 1992, died during a 9-year observation period [10]. The results suggested that introduction of aggressive immunosuppressive therapies containing high-dose corticosteroids and cyclophosphamide has greatly contributed to improvement of clinical outcomes in PAA of BD patients. However, the latest study reported in 2012 revealed the mortality was 26 % (9 of 26 patients), which has not changed since 2004 [7]. Thus, PAA is still one of the most critical prognostic factors, in spite of early diagnosis followed by potent immunosuppressive therapies. Although endovascular intervention, including chemical or coil embolization and surgical operations were tried in some patients [7], they are thought to be optional in an emergency.

Immunosuppressive agents have been shown to be beneficial for venous and cardiac thrombosis and to suppress the recurrence [18, 21, 24, 26, 96].

5.7.2 *Anticoagulation Therapy*

There is a statement regarding anticoagulation in EULAR recommendations as follows [13]:

> Similarly there are no controlled data on, or evidence of benefit from uncontrolled experience with anticoagulants, antiplatelet or antifibrinolytic agents in the management of deep vein thrombosis or for the use of anticoagulation for the arterial lesions of BD.

Rather, the recommendations referred to avoiding these agents in the text due to low incidence of pulmonary embolisms and risk of fatal bleeding from coexisting pulmonary aneurysms [7, 10]. This statement is applicable for the arterial and venous lesions, in both of which coexistence of pulmonary arterial involvement is common. However, because these statements are based on expert opinion rather than evidence, they have to be validated in different countries and different setting as noted in the EULAR recommendations [13].

Although it is hard to differentiate between pulmonary embolism and in situ thrombosis, some investigators think that pulmonary embolism is less likely for the following reasons. First, no pulmonary embolism was reported in a series of postmortem studies in which 130 patients were enrolled [16]. Second, pulmonary arteritis is considered to be the primary underlying pathology [119]. A rim of enhancement at the filling defects in CT scan is consistent with pulmonary artery inflammation rather than pulmonary embolism. Third, anticoagulation without immunosuppressive treatment is ineffective in preventing relapses of BD

[5, 15]. Finally, persistent V/Q mismatch in the ventilation perfusion scintigraphy implies pulmonary vasculitis, unlike thromboembolism in which resolution in time is often the rule [93]. In addition, no studies have shown beneficial effects of anticoagulation on vascular involvement. For these reasons, anticoagulants should be avoided in BD patients.

On the other hand, several reports have supported that anticoagulation therapy is tolerable [3, 8, 18, 19]. Mehta et al. reported that the prevalence of pulmonary embolism was 27.4 % [19]. In their study, 89 % of patients received anticoagulants, whereas bleeding complications were noted in only two patients. Similarly, reports from France and Japan have also shown that anticoagulation for venous thrombosis is not associated with increased risks of fatal pulmonary bleeding, though the beneficial effects have not been statistically proven [3, 8, 18]. In addition to these clinical studies, a study using questionnaires showed that anticoagulants were more frequently used for BD patients with venous and cardiac thrombosis by rheumatologists in Israel and the USA compared to those in Turley [17].

5.7.3 Surgical Operation and Endovascular Intervention

Surgical operations are needed for rupture or impending aneurysm rupture and arterial occlusion in some cases [37, 120–128]. However, the indication should be carefully determined except in emergent cases, because postoperative complications such as graft occlusion, formation of anastomotic psuedoaneurysms, and anastomotic leak are frequent. Relapses of vascular lesions due to BD itself are also common. The complications are sometimes life threatening and require a second operation (Table 5.3). Postoperative complications are thought to be related with underlying vasculitis. The anastomotic fragility may be attributable to weakening of the arterial wall caused by fulminant inflammation. Graft occlusion is also frequently found, presumably due to endothelial dysfunction. Tüzün et al. proposed use of synthetic graft rather than autologous venous graft, in which latent vasculitis might be present, leading to occlusion [37], whereas Koksoy et al. showed no difference in clinical outcomes between PTFE and saphenous vein for interposition [127].

Several studies have shown that concomitant preoperative immunosuppressive therapies decreased postoperative complications [132, 133]. A study has revealed that incidence of prosthetic thrombosis was reduced by use of anticoagulants without increasing bleeding complications [35].

Table 5.3 summarizes the clinical outcomes of surgery and endovascular interventions for arterial involvement in BD patients, suggesting that endovascular intervention can be an alternative in selected cases [121, 126, 128–131]. In addition to low invasion, endovascular therapy may contribute to reducing risk of perioperative complications such as infection under concomitant immunosuppressive therapy. Furthermore, Tekbas et al. have shown that endovascular treatment in addition to conventional pharmacotherapy was effective for DVT in upper extremity central vein and Budd-Chiari syndrome [134].

Table 5.3 Clinical outcomes of surgery and endovascular therapy for arterial involvement in BD patients

	Patients (*n*)	Operation	Mortality (%)	Recurrence (%)	Occlusion (%)	Observation (months)	Reference
Surgery	8	14	13	13	0	82	[120]
	24	24	4	0	17	47	[37]
	3	3	33	0	33	48	[121]
	16	19	0	19	6	17	[122]
	10	30	10	40	0	132	[123]
	20	25	10	50	45	44	[124]
	12	21	17	50	0	45	[125]
	7	8	14	28	0	48	[126]
	23	29	26	24	38	84	[127]
	18	24	6	56	56	12	[128]
Total	141	197	11.3	21.3	19.3		
Endovascular therapy	7	8	0	14.3	28.6	28	[129]
	9	11	0	22.2	22.2	24	[130]
	2	2	0	0	0	33	[121]
	10	12	10	20	0	25.8	[131]
	16	20	0	12.5	12.5	48	[126]
	10	10	0	0	20	12	[128]
Total	54	63	3.7	11.1	9.5		

5.7.4 *Biologic Agents*

In Japan, infliximab has been used as a standard therapy for uveitis of BD patients since 2007, whereas adalimumab has been authorized for the intestinal lesions since 2013. Beneficial effects of infliximab have been reported in BD patients with serious forms of vascular lesions such as PAA, deep vein thrombosis, aortic dissection, and arterial aneurysms [77, 135–140]. Similarly, a case report showed efficacy of adalimumab for PAA [141]. Clinical trials with infliximab for vasculo-BD patients are now undergoing in Japan.

5.8 Summary

Vascular lesions cause diverse clinical manifestations in BD patients, and some of them including PAA, peripheral arterial aneurysms, and Budd-Chiari syndrome can be fatal. Although immunosuppression is essential for the treatment, it is uncertain whether anticoagulation is beneficial or not. Although surgical operations are required in some patients, postoperative complications are frequent and can be fatal. Concomitant immunosuppressive therapy is not only effective for the disease itself but also helpful for reducing postoperative complications and improving clinical outcomes. Biologics, especially TNF inhibitors, are promising as a therapeutic option for vascular involvement as well as uveitis and intestinal involvement of BD.

References

1. Sakane T, et al. Behçet's disease. N Engl J Med. 1999;341(17):1284–91.
2. International Study Group for Behçet's Disease. Criteria for diagnosis of Behçet's disease. Lancet. 1990;335(8697):1078–80.
3. Ideguchi H, et al. Characteristics of vascular involvement in Behçet's disease in Japan: a retrospective cohort study. Clin Exp Rheumatol. 2011;29(4 Suppl 67):S47–53.
4. Jennette JC, et al. 2012 revised International Chapel Hill Consensus Conference Nomenclature of Vasculitides. Arthritis Rheum. 2013;65(1):1–11.
5. Uzun O, et al. Pulmonary vasculitis in Behçet disease: a cumulative analysis. Chest. 2005;127(6):2243–53.
6. Uzun O, et al. Pulmonary involvement in Behçet's disease. Respiration. 2008;75(3):310–21.
7. Seyahi E, et al. Pulmonary artery involvement and associated lung disease in Behçet disease: a series of 47 patients. Medicine. 2012;91(1):35–48.
8. Saadoun D, et al. Long-term outcome of arterial lesions in Behçet disease: a series of 101 patients. Medicine. 2012;91(1):18–24.
9. Saadoun D, et al. Mortality in Behcet's disease. Arthritis Rheum. 2010;62:2806–12.
10. Hamuryudan V, et al. Pulmonary artery aneurysms in Behçet syndrome. Am J Med. 2004;117(11):867–70.
11. Kural-Seyahi E, et al. The long-term mortality and morbidity of Behcet syndrome: a 2-decade outcome survey of 387 patients followed at a dedicated center. Medicine. 2003; 82(1):60–76.
12. Hamuryudan V, et al. Pulmonary arterial aneurysms in Behçet's syndrome: a report of 24 cases. Br J Rheumatol. 1994;33(1):48–51.
13. Hatemi G, EULAR Expert Committee, et al. EULAR recommendations for the management of Behçet disease. Ann Rheum Dis. 2008;67(12):1656–62.
14. Hatemi G, et al. Management of Behçet disease: a systematic literature review for the European League Against Rheumatism evidence-based recommendations for the management of Behçet disease. Ann Rheum Dis. 2009;68(10):1528–34.
15. Ahn JK, et al. Treatment of venous thrombosis associated with Behcet's disease: immunosuppressive therapy alone versus immunosuppressive therapy plus anticoagulation. Clin Rheumatol. 2008;27(2):201–5.
16. Lakhanpal S, et al. Pathologic features of Behçet's syndrome: a review of Japanese autopsy registry data. Hum Pathol. 1985;16(8):790–5.
17. Tayer-Shifman OE, et al. Major vessel thrombosis in Behçet's disease: the dilemma of anticoagulant therapy – the approach of rheumatologists from different countries. Clin Exp Rheumatol. 2012;30(5):735–40.
18. Desbois AC, et al. Immunosuppressants reduce venous thrombosis relapse in Behçet's disease. Arthritis Rheum. 2012;64(8):2753–60.
19. Mehta P, Laffan M, Haskard DO. Thrombosis and Behçet's syndrome in non-endemic regions. Rheumatology (Oxford). 2010;49(11):2003–4.
20. Ideguchi H, et al. Neurological manifestations of Behçet's disease in Japan: a study of 54 patients. J Neurol. 2010;257(6):1012–20.
21. Koc Y, et al. Vascular involvement in Behçet's disease. J Rheumatol. 1992;19(3):402–10.
22. al-Dalaan AN, et al. Behcet's disease in Saudi Arabia. J Rheumatol. 1994;21(4):658–61.
23. Gurler A, et al. Clinical manifestations of Behçet's disease: an analysis of 2147 patients. Yonsei Med J. 1997;38(6):423–7.

24. Tohmé A, et al. Vascular manifestations of Behçet's disease. Eighteen cases among 140 patients. Joint Bone Spine. 2003;70(5):384–9.
25. Düzgün N, et al. Characteristics of vascular involvement in Behçet's disease. Scand J Rheumatol. 2006;35(1):65–8.
26. Sarica-Kucukoglu R, et al. Vascular involvement in Behçet's disease: a retrospective analysis of 2319 cases. Int J Dermatol. 2006;45(8):919–21.
27. Zhang Z, et al. Behcet's disease seen in China: analysis of 334 cases. Rheumatol Int. 2013;33(3):645–8.
28. Yazici H, et al. Influence of age of onset and patient's sex on the prevalence and severity of manifestations of Behçet's syndrome. Ann Rheum Dis. 1984;43(6):783–9.
29. Hamza M. Large artery involvement in Behçet's disease. J Rheumatol. 1987;14(3):554–9.
30. Calamia KT, et al. Major vessel involvement in Behçet disease. Curr Opin Rheumatol. 2005;17(1):1–8.
31. Alli N, et al. Patient characteristics in Behçet disease: a retrospective analysis of 213 Turkish patients during 2001-4. Am J Clin Dermatol. 2009;10(6):411–8.
32. Yazici H, et al. The combined use of HLA-B5 and the pathergy test as diagnostic markers of Behçet's disease in Turkey. J Rheumatol. 1980;7(2):206–10.
33. Saadoun D, et al. Cerebral venous thrombosis in Behçet's disease. Arthritis Rheum. 2009;61(4):518–26.
34. Miyamoto N, et al. Estrogen protects against cellular infiltration by reducing the expressions of E-selectin and IL-6 in endotoxin-induced uveitis. J Immunol. 1999;163(1):374–9.
35. Lê Thi Huong D, et al. Arterial lesions in Behçet's disease. A study in 25 patients. J Rheumatol. 1995;22(11):2103–13.
36. Ko GY, et al. The vascular manifestations of Behçet's disease: angiographic and CT findings. Br J Radiol. 2000;73(876):1270–4.
37. Tüzün H, et al. Management of aneurysms in Behçet's syndrome: an analysis of 24 patients. Surgery. 1997;121(2):150–6.
38. Kobayashi M, et al. Neutrophil and endothelial cell activation in the vasa vasorum in vasculo-Behçet disease. Histopathology. 2000;36(4):362–71.
39. Suzuki K, et al. Emergency operation for distal aortic arch aneurysm in Behcet's disease. Jpn J Thorac Cardiovasc Surg. 2005;53(7):389–92.
40. Marzban M, et al. Cardiac and great vessel involvement in "Behcet's disease". J Card Surg. 2008;23(6):765–8.
41. Hoffman GS. Large-vessel vasculitis: unresolved issues. Arthritis Rheum. 2003; 48(9):2406–14.
42. Ucer E, et al. Uncommon presentation of Behçet's syndrome: aortic aneurysm and dissection due to Behçet's syndrome. Acta Cardiol. 2006;61(3):356–8.
43. Suzuki A, et al. Surgical consideration of aortitis involving the aortic root. Circulation. 1989;80(3 Pt 1):I222–32.
44. Reus M, et al. Treatment of a radial artery pseudoaneurysm with ultrasound-guided percutaneous thrombin injection in a patient with Behçet's syndrome. J Clin Ultrasound. 2003;31(8):440–4.
45. Freyrie A, et al. True and false aneurysms in Behçet's disease: case report with ultrastructural observations. J Vasc Surg. 1993;17(4):762–7.
46. Kingston M, et al. Aneurysm after arterial puncture in Behçet's disease. Br Med J. 1979;1(6180):1766–7.
47. Ugurlu S, et al. Prevalence of angina, myocardial infarction and intermittent claudication assessed by Rose Questionnaire among patients with Behcet's syndrome. Rheumatology (Oxford). 2008;47(4):472–5.
48. Sagduyu A, et al. An unusual case of Behçet's disease presenting with bilateral internal carotid artery occlusion. J Neurol Neurosurg Psychiatry. 2002;73(3):343.
49. Cakmak HA, Erturk E, et al. The rare complication of Behcet's syndrome: concomitance of coronary slow flow with acute coronary syndrome. BMJ Case Rep. 2012;2012. doi:10.1136/bcr-2012-006388.

50. Ergelen M, et al. Management of acute coronary syndrome in a case of Behçet's disease. Blood Coagul Fibrinolysis. 2009;20(8):715–8.
51. Jin SJ, et al. Acute myocardial infarction due to sinus of Valsalva aneurysm in a patient with Behçet's disease. Clin Exp Rheumatol. 2008;26(4 Suppl 50):S117–20.
52. Arishiro K, et al. Vascular Behçet's disease with coronary artery aneurysm. Intern Med. 2006;45(15):903–7.
53. Tezcan H, et al. Coronary stent implantation in Behçet's disease. Clin Exp Rheumatol. 2002;20(5):704–6.
54. Schirmer M, et al. Valvular disease and myocardial infarctions in a patient with Behçet disease. J Clin Rheumatol. 2003;9(5):316–20.
55. Trad S, et al. 18F-fluorodeoxyglucose-positron emission tomography scanning is a useful tool for therapy evaluation of arterial aneurysm in Behçet's disease. Joint Bone Spine. 2013;80(4):420–3.
56. Cho SB, et al. Detection of cardiovascular system involvement in Behçet's disease using fluorodeoxyglucose positron emission tomography. Semin Arthritis Rheum. 2011;40(5):461–6.
57. Lee KH, et al. The role of (18) F-fluorodeoxyglucose-positron emission tomography in the assessment of disease activity in patients with Takayasu arteritis. Arthritis Rheum. 2012;64(3):866–75.
58. Kuzu MA, et al. Vascular involvement in Behçet's disease: 8-year audit. World J Surg. 1994;18(6):948–53; discussion 953-4.
59. Tursen U, et al. Evaluation of clinical findings according to sex in 2313 Turkish patients with Behçet's disease. Int J Dermatol. 2003;42(5):346–51.
60. Ames PR, et al. Thrombosis in Behçet's disease: a retrospective survey from a single UK centre. Rheumatology (Oxford). 2001;40(6):652–5.
61. White RH, et al. Effect of ethnicity and gender on the incidence of venous thromboembolism in a diverse population in California in 1996. Thromb Haemost. 2005;93(2):298–305.
62. Mok CC, et al. Incidence and risk factors of thromboembolism in systemic lupus erythematosus: a comparison of three ethnic groups. Arthritis Rheum. 2005;52(9):2774–82.
63. Bertina RM, et al. Mutation in blood coagulation factor v associated with resistance to activated protein c. Nature. 1994;369(6475):64–7.
64. Svensson PJ, Dahlback B. Resistance to activated protein c as a basis for venous thrombosis. N Engl J Med. 1994;330(8):517–22.
65. Margaglione M, et al. Increased risk for venous thrombosis in carriers of the prothrombin g-->a20210 gene variant. Ann Intern Med. 1998;129(2):89–93.
66. Ricart JM, et al. Thrombophilic risk factors and homocysteine levels in Behçet's disease in eastern Spain and their association with thrombotic events. Thromb Haemost. 2006;95(4):618–24.
67. Silingardi M, et al. Factor v Leiden and prothrombin gene g20210a mutations in Italian patients with Behçet's disease and deep vein thrombosis. Arthritis Rheum. 2004;51(2):177–83.
68. Espinosa G, et al. Vascular involvement in Behçet's disease: relation with thrombophilic factors, coagulation activation, and thrombomodulin. Am J Med. 2002;112(1):37–43.
69. Leiba M, et al. Thrombophilic factors are not the leading cause of thrombosis in Behçet's disease. Ann Rheum Dis. 2004;63(11):1445–9.
70. Chambers JC, et al. Vascular endothelial function and oxidative stress mechanisms in patients with Behçet's syndrome. J Am Coll Cardiol. 2001;37(2):517–20.
71. Oh SH, et al. Dermatological features in Behçet disease-associated vena cava obstruction. Br J Dermatol. 2008;159(3):555–60.
72. Zhang L, et al. Chylothorax and chylopericardium in Behçet's diseases: case report and literature review. Clin Rheumatol. 2013;32(7):1107–11.
73. Benjilali L, et al. Chylothorax and chylopericardium in a young man with Behçet's disease. Joint Bone Spine. 2008;75(6):743–5.
74. Oh SH, et al. Dermatological features in Behçet disease-associated vena cava obstruction. Br J Dermatol. 2008;159(3):555–60.

75. Ben Ghorbel I, et al. Budd-Chiari syndrome associated with Behçet's disease. Gastroenterol Clin Biol. 2008;32(3):316–20.
76. Bayraktar Y, et al. Budd-Chiari syndrome: a common complication of Behçet's disease. Am J Gastroenterol. 1997;92(5):858–62.
77. Seyahi E, et al. Infliximab in the treatment of hepatic vein thrombosis (Budd-Chiari syndrome) in three patients with Behcet's syndrome. Rheumatology (Oxford). 2007;46(7):1213–4.
78. Tunc R, et al. Cerebral venous thrombosis is associated with major vessel disease in Behçet's syndrome. Ann Rheum Dis. 2004;63(12):1693–4.
79. Akman-Demir G, et al. Clinical patterns of neurological involvement in Behçet's disease: evaluation of 200 patients. The Neuro-Behçet Study Group. Brain. 1999;122(Pt 11):2171–82.
80. Wechsler B, et al. Cerebral venous thrombosis in Behçet's disease: clinical study and long-term follow-up of 25 cases. Neurology. 1992;42(3 Pt 1):614–8.
81. Tuthill JI, Khamashta MA. Management of antiphospholipid syndrome. J Autoimmun. 2009;33(2):92–8.
82. Tan VP, et al. Venous and arterial disease in inflammatory bowel disease. J Gastroenterol Hepatol. 2013;28(7):1095–113.
83. Nanke Y, et al. Cryptogenic organizing pneumonia in two patients with Behçet's disease. Clin Exp Rheumatol. 2007;25(4 Suppl 45):S103–6.
84. Ning-Sheng L, et al. Bronchiolitis obliterans organizing pneumonia in a patient with Behçet's disease. Scand J Rheumatol. 2004;33(6):437–40.
85. Gül A, et al. Organizing pneumonia associated with pulmonary artery aneurysms in Behçet's disease. Rheumatology (Oxford). 1999;38(12):1285–9.
86. Emad Y, et al. Hughes-Stovin syndrome: is it incomplete Behçet's? Report of two cases and review of the literature. Clin Rheumatol. 2007;26(11):1993–6.
87. Erkan D, et al. Is Hughes-Stovin syndrome Behçet's disease? Clin Exp Rheumatol. 2004;22(4 Suppl 34):S64–8.
88. Bowman S, Honey M. Pulmonary arterial occlusions and aneurysms: a forme fruste of Behçet's or Hughes-Stovin syndrome. Br Heart J. 1990;63(1):66–8.
89. Tunaci A, et al. Thoracic involvement in Behçet's disease: pathologic, clinical, and imaging features. AJR Am J Roentgenol. 1995;164(1):51–6.
90. Ceylan N, et al. Pulmonary and vascular manifestations of Behcet disease: imaging findings. AJR Am J Roentgenol. 2010;194(2):W158–64.
91. Hiller N, et al. Thoracic manifestations of Behçet disease at CT. Radiographics. 2004;24(3):801–8.
92. Basoglu T, et al. Bilateral pulmonary artery aneurysms in a patient with Behcet syndrome: evaluation with radionuclide angiography and V/Q lung scanning. Clin Nucl Med. 1998;23(11):735–8.
93. Caglar M, et al. 99Tcm-MAA lung scintigraphy in patients with Behçet's disease: its value and correlation with clinical course and other diagnostic modalities. Nucl Med Commun. 2000;21(2):171–9.
94. Loh H, et al. Pulmonary artery aneurysm with false-positive FDG PET in a patient with Behcet disease. Clin Nucl Med. 2010;35(4):286–8.
95. Denecke T, et al. PET/CT visualises inflammatory activity of pulmonary artery aneurysms in Behçet disease. Eur J Nucl Med Mol Imaging. 2007;34(6):970.
96. Geri G, et al. Spectrum of cardiac lesions in Behçet disease: a series of 52 patients and review of the literature. Medicine. 2012;91(1):25–34.
97. Atzeni F, et al. Behçet's disease and cardiovascular involvement. Lupus. 2005;14(9):723–6.
98. Türkölmez S, et al. Evaluation of myocardial perfusion in patients with Behçet's disease. Ann Nucl Med. 2005;19(3):201–6.
99. Vaiopoulos G, et al. Asymptomatic pericarditis in Adamantiadis-Behçet's disease. Clin Exp Rheumatol. 1995;13(5):649–51.

100. Tahir T. A case of acute constrictive pericarditis associated with Behçet's disease. Int J Rheum Dis. 2011;14(4):e51–3.
101. Nojiri C, et al. Conduction disturbance in Behçet's disease. Association with ruptured aneurysm of the sinus of valsalva into the left ventricular cavity. Chest. 1984;86(4):636–8.
102. Yu JS, et al. Rapidly progressive cardiac manifestation of Behçet's disease involving conduction system and aortic valve. J Cardiovasc Ultrasound. 2011;19(4):199–202.
103. Gürgün C, et al. Cardiovascular involvement in Behçet's disease. Jpn Heart J. 2002;43(4):389–98.
104. Han JK, et al. Behçet's disease as a frequently unrecognized cause of aortic regurgitation: suggestive and misleading echocardiography findings. J Am Soc Echocardiogr. 2009;22(11):1269–74.
105. Liang MY, et al. Surgical technique for aortic regurgitation attributable to Behcet's disease: modified aortic valve replacement with reinforcement of the aortic wall. Eur J Cardiothorac Surg. 2012;41(3):647–8.d.
106. Ma WG, et al. Aortic regurgitation caused by Behçet's disease: surgical experience during an 11-year period. J Card Surg. 2012;27(1):39–44.
107. Song JK, et al. Factors determining outcomes of aortic valve surgery in patients with aortic regurgitation due to Behçet's disease: impact of preoperative echocardiographic features. J Am Soc Echocardiogr. 2011;24(9):995–1003.
108. Azuma T, et al. Aortic valve replacement in Behcet's disease: surgical modification to prevent valve detachment. Eur J Cardiothorac Surg. 2009;36(4):771–2.
109. Jeong DS, et al. Long-term experience of surgical treatment for aortic regurgitation attributable to Behçet's disease. Ann Thorac Surg. 2009;87(6):1775–82.
110. Lee I, et al. Cardiac Behçet disease presenting as aortic valvulitis/aortitis or right heart inflammatory mass: a clinicopathologic study of 12 cases. Am J Surg Pathol. 2008;32(3):390–8.
111. Binak K, et al. Left ventricular aneurysm and acute pericarditis in a case of Behcet's disease. J Rheumatol. 1980;7(4):578–80.
112. Di Eusanio G, et al. Left ventricular aneurysm secondary to Behçet's disease. Ann Thorac Surg. 1991;51(1):131–2.
113. Zhuang J, et al. Acute myocardial infarction and ascending aortic aneurysm in a child with Behçet's disease. Turk J Pediatr. 2008;50(1):81–5.
114. Yue C, et al. Cardiac mass in Behçet's disease. Clin Exp Rheumatol. 2012;30(3 Suppl 72):S27–31.
115. Sacré K, et al. Unusual cardiovascular events in Behçet's disease. Clin Exp Rheumatol. 2010;28(4 Suppl 60):S82–5.
116. Huong DL, et al. Endomyocardial fibrosis in Behçet's disease. Ann Rheum Dis. 1997;56(3):205–8.
117. Zhu YL, et al. The clinical characteristics and outcome of intracardiac thrombus and aortic valvular involvement in Behçet's disease: an analysis of 20 cases. Clin Exp Rheumatol. 2012;30(3 Suppl 72):S40–5. Epub 2012 Sep 25. PubMed PMID: 23010261.
118. Piga M, et al. Successful thrombolytic therapy for recurrent right ventricular thrombosis in Behçet's disease. Clin Exp Rheumatol. 2010;28(4 Suppl 60):S76–8.
119. Hamuryudan V, et al. The menacing pulmonary artery aneurysms of Behçet's syndrome. Clin Exp Rheumatol. 2004;22(4 Suppl 34):S1–3.
120. Okada K, et al. Surgical management of Behçet's aortitis: a report of eight patients. Ann Thorac Surg. 1997;64(1):116–9.
121. Nitecki SS, et al. Abdominal aortic aneurysm in Behçet's disease: new treatment options for an old and challenging problem. Isr Med Assoc J. 2004;6(3):152–5.
122. Kalko Y, et al. The surgical treatment of arterial aneurysms in Behçet disease: a report of 16 patients. J Vasc Surg. 2005;42(4):673–7.
123. Hosaka A, et al. Long-term outcome after surgical treatment of arterial lesions in Behçet disease. J Vasc Surg. 2005;42(1):116–21.

124. Iscan ZH, et al. Compelling nature of arterial manifestations in Behcet disease. J Vasc Surg. 2005;41(1):53–8.
125. Kwon TW, et al. Surgical treatment result of abdominal aortic aneurysm in Behçet's disease. Eur J Vasc Endovasc Surg. 2008;35(2):173–80.
126. Kim WH, et al. Effectiveness and safety of endovascular aneurysm treatment in patients with vasculo-Behçet disease. J Endovasc Ther. 2009;16(5):631–6.
127. Koksoy C, et al. Surgical treatment of peripheral aneurysms in patients with Behcet's disease. Eur J Vasc Endovasc Surg. 2011;42(4):525–30.
128. Yang SS, et al. Peripheral arterial involvement in Behcet's disease: an analysis of the results from a Korean referral center. Rheumatol Int. 2013;33(8):2101–8.
129. Park JH, et al. Aortic and arterial aneurysms in Behçet disease: management with stent-grafts–initial experience. Radiology. 2001;220(3):745–50.
130. Kwon Koo B, et al. Endovascular therapy combined with immunosuppressive treatment for pseudoaneurysms in patients with Behçet's disease. J Endovasc Ther. 2003;10(1):75–80.
131. Liu CW, et al. Endovascular treatment of aortic pseudoaneurysm in Behçet disease. J Vasc Surg. 2009;50(5):1025–30.
132. Park MC, et al. Surgical outcomes and risk factors for postoperative complications in patients with Behcet's disease. Clin Rheumatol. 2007;26(9):1475–80.
133. Ha YJ, et al. Long-term clinical outcomes and risk factors for the occurrence of post-operative complications after cardiovascular surgery in patients with Behçet's disease. Clin Exp Rheumatol. 2012;30(3 Suppl 72):S18–26.
134. Tekbas G, et al. Endovascular treatment of veno-occlusive Behcet's disease. Cardiovasc Intervent Radiol. 2012;35(4):826–31.
135. Adler S, et al. Behçet's disease: successful treatment with infliximab in 7 patients with severe vascular manifestations. A retrospective analysis. Arthritis Care Res. 2012;64(4):607–11.
136. Tolosa-Vilella C, et al. Infliximab for life-threatening pulmonary artery aneurysms in Behçet's disease. A case report. Clin Exp Rheumatol. 2011;29(4 Suppl 67):S94–5.
137. Schreiber BE, et al. Resolution of Behçet's syndrome associated pulmonary arterial aneurysms with infliximab. Semin Arthritis Rheum. 2011;41(3):482–7.
138. Baki K, et al. Behcet's disease with life-threatening haemoptoe and pulmonary aneurysms: complete remission after infliximab treatment. Ann Rheum Dis. 2006;65(11):1531–2.
139. Yoshida S, et al. Good response to infliximab in a patient with deep vein thrombosis associated with Behçet disease. Mod Rheumatol. 2012;22(5):791–5.
140. Rokutanda R, et al. Infliximab for Behçet disease with aortic involvement: two novel case reports without concurrent use of immunosuppressive agents or corticosteroids. Mod Rheumatol. 2013;23(2):412–3.
141. Lee SW, Lee SY, Kim KN, Jung JK, Chung WT. Adalimumab treatment for life threatening pulmonary artery aneurysm in Behçet disease: a case report. Clin Rheumatol. 2010; 29(1):91–3.

Chapter 6
Neurological Involvement

Shunsei Hirohata

Abstract Neuro-Behçet's disease (NB) is one of the difficult complications of Behçet's disease (BD), consisting of acute type and chronic progressive type. Diagnostic criteria for both types of NB have been recently established based on the results of a multicenter retrospective survey on BD patients with neurological manifestations in Japan. Administration of corticosteroids is usually necessary and effective in attacks of acute NB, although they are sometimes self-limiting. In addition, infliximab and interferon alpha might also be effective during the attacks in acute NB. Recent studies have disclosed that colchicine as well as cessation of cyclosporin A (CyA) if used at the attacks is effective for preventing the recurrence of further attacks of acute NB. As to chronic progressive NB, one should keep in mind that corticosteroids, cyclophosphamide, and azathioprine are not effective at all. Low-dose methotrexate (MTX) has been shown to decrease cerebrospinal fluid IL-6 levels without progression of neuropsychological manifestations and is now a gold-standard treatment. Recent studies have demonstrated that infliximab has a beneficial effect in chronic progressive NB patients with inadequate responses to MTX.

Keywords Methotrexate • MRI • Infliximab • Cerebrospinal fluid • IL-6

6.1 Introduction

Behçet's disease (BD) is an inflammatory disease, characterized by aphthous stomatitis, uveitis, genital ulcers, and skin lesions, including acne-like pustulosis, erythema nodosum, and superficial thrombophlebitis. In general, the patients present recurrent episodes of remission and exacerbation of these symptoms, whereas chronic sustained inflammation in certain tissues is rare [1]. Although the association with certain genetic factors has been demonstrated, its etiology still remains unclear. Of note, there are common characteristic histopathological features in the inflamed tissues, such as perivascular cuffing of mononuclear cells and polymorph

S. Hirohata, M.D. (✉)
Department of Rheumatology and Infectious Diseases, Kitasato University School of Medicine, 1-15-1 Kitasato, Minami-ku, Sagamihara, Kanagawa 252-0374, Japan
e-mail: shunsei_tenpoint@yahoo.co.jp

Y. Ishigatsubo (ed.), *Behçet's Disease*,
DOI 10.1007/978-4-431-54487-6_6

nuclear leukocytes, and thrombophilia or thrombophlebilis involving mainly small and large veins. In these regard, BD is different from other vasculitides and has been classified as variable vessel vasculitis in 2012 Chapel Hill consensus conference [2].

Posterior uveitis is one of the most serious complications of BD, which usually results in the loss of vision and therefore seriously affects the activity of daily life of the patients. In addition, vascular involvement, intestinal involvement, and neurological involvement are usually life threatening and thus require intensive treatment [1].

Neurological involvement in BD is either caused by primary neural parenchymal lesions (neuro-Behçet's disease (NB)) or is secondary to major vascular involvement, such as cerebral venous thrombosis (CVT) [3, 4]. CVT in BD is rarely complicated with the parenchymal lesions with a better prognosis compared with NB [3] and should therefore be regarded as vasculo-Behçet's disease [3]. Notably, the incidence of CVT is quite low in Japan compared with other countries, including Turkey [4, 5].

In NB, involvement of the brainstem is the most common, whereas spinal cord lesions, cerebral hemispheric lesions, and meningeal lesions also take place [6–8]. The etiology and pathogenesis of NB remain unclear. Most patients with NB present only a single attack, whereas one-third of patients repeat further attacks [6–8]. On the other hand, a number of studies have disclosed the presence of patients who underwent progressive deterioration leading to disability either with or without a history of previous attacks, thus called as primary or secondary progression [6–8]. Nonetheless, factors determining prognosis, reliable diagnostic tools, and appropriate treatment regimens have not been delineated until recent periods of time.

Accumulating efforts have successfully clarified that NB can be classified into acute type (acute NB) and chronic progressive type (chronic progressive NB) depending on their differential clinical courses, especially on their differential responses to steroids [9–11]. Thus, acute NB responds well to corticosteroid and is usually self-limiting. By contrast, chronic progressive NB is characterized by intractable neurobehavior changes and ataxia, which progress in spite of high doses of steroids or immunosuppressants such as azathioprine or cyclophosphamide [9–11]. Of note, it has been found that methotrexate (MTX) is effective for CP NB [10, 11]. In addition, increasing attention has been paid to the effect of antitumor necrosis factor alpha (TNF-α) therapy in BD, including NB [1]. The present article overviews an update on the pathogenesis, clinical manifestation, diagnosis, and treatment of NB and introduces new guidelines for diagnosis and treatment of NB, which have been recently established through multicenter epidemiological studies in Japan [5].

6.2 Clinical Manifestations

6.2.1 Cerebral Venous Thrombosis (CVT)

CVT has been found to occur in 10–20 % of BD patients with neurological involvement [8, 11–13]. CVT is characterized by thrombosis of the venous sinuses, especially superior sagittal sinus, leading to increased intracranial pressure with headache, papilledema, cranial nerve palsies, and mental changes [8, 11–13]. CVT in BD usually occurs relatively slowly, but acute onset of seizures and focal neurological symptoms is sometimes seen [14]. The occurrence of CVT together with primary central nervous system (CNS) parenchymal lesions in the same patient is rare [11, 13, 15]. CVT in BD is frequently associated with systemic major vessel disease, such as venous thrombosis of large vessels, and sometimes pulmonary artery aneurysm and should therefore be regarded as vasculo-Behçet's disease [13, 16, 17]. Overall, patients with CVT have a better neurological prognosis than those with neuroparenchymal NB. Thus, recurrence of CVT and persistent neurological deficits are less likely to occur. However, due to the increased association with major systemic vessel disease, patients with CVT may not be always associated with a favorable outcome, especially in case they are complicated with pulmonary artery aneurysm [7].

In the Japanese multicenter retrospective cohort study of BD patients who presented neurological manifestations between 1988 and 2008, only 1 of the 144 patients showed cerebral CVT, confirming that the incidence of CVT in Japan is much lower than that in the Middle East or European countries [2, 5–8]. The reason for the paucity of CVT in Japan remains unclear. In this regard, the frequency of vasculo-Behçet's disease is lower in Japan [18]. By contrast, the frequency of intestinal involvement is much more common in Japanese BD patients [1]. It is therefore suggested that some ethnic differences in genetic factors might be involved.

6.2.2 Parenchymal Involvement (Neuro-Behçet's Disease [NB])

6.2.2.1 General Remarks

The brainstem-diencephalon and pontobulbar regions are most frequently involved in NB [2]. Subsequently, motor symptoms, cerebellar symptoms, brainstem symptoms, and dysarthria are often presented [7]. It should be emphasized, however, that behavioral symptoms are seen in approximately 10 %. Although headache is the most common symptom in NB [7, 19], it can occur in BD patients independent of the neurological involvement [16]. As to the neurological signs, it is noteworthy that pyramidal tract signs are frequently observed even in the absence of apparent motor dysfunctions [2, 6].

The differential diagnosis of NB includes many neurological diseases. Among miscellaneous diseases, multiple sclerosis has been one of the leading misdiagnoses of BD due to the similarity in preference for lesions. The major lesion is located in the brainstem-diencephalon-basal ganglion region on magnetic resonance imaging (MRI) scans in NB [8]. However, in some cases, the predominant lesion may be found in the periventricular white matter, mimicking the lesions found in multiple sclerosis. In such cases, cerebrospinal fluid (CSF) pleocytosis with elevation of polymorphonuclear cells [8], the absence of more than 2 oligoclonal IgG bands [9], and the elevation of CSF IL-6 [1] may favor the diagnosis of NB. When patients of BD present neurological manifestations, differential diagnosis should include isolated headache syndromes, cardiogenic embolic stroke, brain tumors, and syringomyelia [7]. In addition to careful neurological examination, the evaluation of CSF and MRI scans is mandatory.

Accumulating evidence has demonstrated that NB can be classified into acute type and chronic progressive type based upon clinical courses and responses to treatment [5, 9]. Accordingly, Akman-Demir et al. disclosed that patients with NB have different clinical courses, including attack(s) and remission, secondary progression, primary progression, and silent neurological involvement [8]. Attack(s) and remission in their series are the same as acute type, whereas primary and secondary progression corresponds to chronic progressive type in our classification [5, 9]. Notably, most of our patients with chronic progressive NB had preceding history of acute neurological events [5, 9]. It is also likely that silent neurological involvement might be a modest form of acute NB and be regarded as preceding symptoms of primary progressive courses [5, 8, 9].

6.2.2.2 Acute NB

Acute NB is characterized by attacks of inflammatory lesions in brain parenchyma and/or meningens, detected as high-intensity areas in T2-weighted images or fluid-attenuated inversion recovery (FLAIR) images on MRI scans [5] (Fig. 6.1). Although rare, the spinal cord can be involved. Patients usually present focal neurological deficits. Among a variety of neurological manifestations, headache and fever are the most common in acute NB (Table 6.1) [5]. Acute attacks respond well to corticosteroid therapy and are usually self-limiting, although recurrence sometimes takes place. It should be noted, however, that severe neurological lesions can lead to permanent damage or disability in spite of extensive treatment [7, 8, 20]. Of note, cyclosporin A (CyA) is frequency associated with the development of acute neurological attacks, which are considered to be a subtype of acute NB [21].

6.2.2.3 Chronic Progressive NB

Chronic progressive NB is characterized by intractable, slowly progressive neurobehavior changes regardless of neurological deficits, leading to severe disability and deterioration [1, 7]. Progressive neurobehavioral manifestations include ataxia, dysarthria, urinary incontinence, and neuropsychological symptoms in chronic progressive NB (Table 6.1) [5, 9]. The progressive neuropsychological symptoms are cognitive dysfunction, euphoria, loss of insight, disinhibition, indifference to their disease, psychomotor agitation, or retardation, with paranoid attitudes and obsessive concerns [7]. These symptoms should not be confused with psychosis associated with the use of corticosteroid or other therapy.

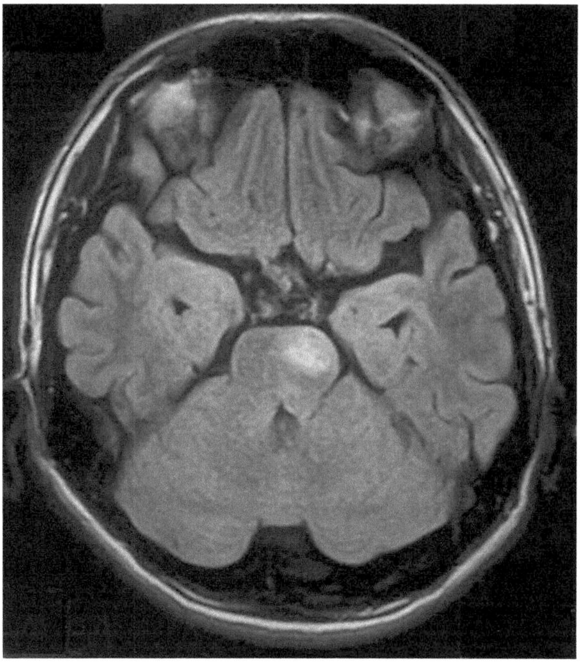

Fig. 6.1 Axial fluid attenuated inversion recovery (FLAIR) brain MRI of a patient with acute NB, showing high-density lesions in the left pons

Table 6.1 Clinical symptoms in 144 patients with BS

	Acute NB	Chronic progressive NB	Non-NB	*p* value*
n	76	35	33	
Headache	41 (53.9 %)	2 (5.7 %)	14 (42.4 %)	<0.0001
Fever	43 (56.6 %)	1 (2.9 %)	3 (9.1 %)	<0.0001
Neurobehavior/cognitive symptoms	7 (9.2 %)	18 (51.4 %)	3 (9.1 %)	<0.0001
Alteration of consciousness	7 (9.2 %)	1 (2.9 %)	5 (15.1 %)	0.2088
Ataxia	9 (11.8 %)	17 (48.6 %)	10 (30.3 %)	0.0001
Dysarthria	14 (18.4 %)	15 (42.9 %)	3 (9.1 %)	0.0019
Focal symptoms (motor, sensory, etc.)	20 (26.3 %)	7 (20.0 %)	10 (30.3 %)	0.6136
Bladder bowel disturbances	2 (2.6 %)	6 (17.1 %)	2 (6.1 %)	0.0208
Dizziness	0	2 (5.7 %)	4 (12.1 %)	0.0123
Vertigo	8 (10.5 %)	0	3 (9.1 %)	0.1429

From Ref. [5]
*Statistical significance was evaluated by chi-square test

One of the most important features in chronic progressive NB is marked persistent elevation of CSF IL-6 (>20 pg/ml) despite a modest increase in cell numbers and total protein [9]. The characteristic findings on MRI include atrophy of the brainstem and cerebellum, but not high-intensity lesions in FLAIR images, in chronic progressive NB (Fig. 6.2). Although cerebral atrophy is also seen, brainstem atrophy is more remarkable and specific for chronic progressive NB.

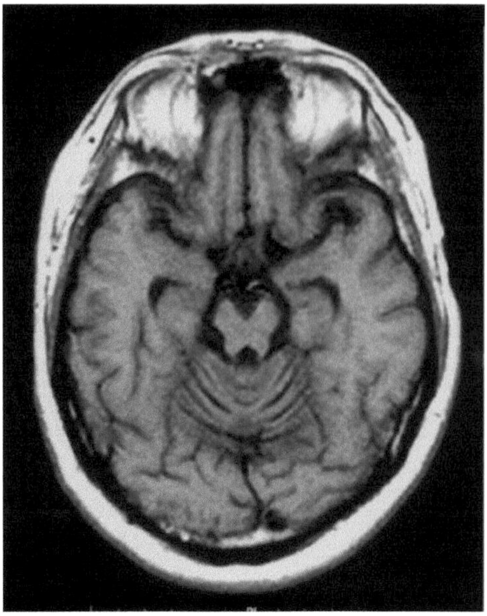

Fig. 6.2 Axial fluid-attenuated inversion recovery (FLAIR) brain MRI of a patient with chronic progressive type neuro-Behçet's syndrome, showing atrophy of the midbrain

Most patients (approximately 90 %) in our series with chronic progressive NB were HLA-B51-positive, who had history of attacks of acute NB before the development of progressive neuropsychological symptoms [9]. In this regard, it has been revealed that HLA-B51 and cigarette smoking, and especially their combination, are risk factors for chronic progressive NB [22]. It is likely that certain substances in cigarettes might be immunogenic in the context of HLA-B51, resulting in the persistent stimulation of immune responses within the central nervous system (CNS) in NB [22]. Of note, chronic progressive NB is resistant to conventional treatment with corticosteroid, with cyclophosphamide, or with azathioprine [9, 23]. Instead, we have disclosed that low-dose weekly MTX has beneficial effects in the treatment of chronic progressive NB [20], as will be discussed later.

6.2.2.4 Acute NB During the Course of Chronic Progressive NB (Acute on Chronic)

It remained uncertain whether acute NB and chronic progressive NB might be independent clinical entities or represent different stages of the disease. In fact, some patients with chronic progressive NB have preceding histories of acute NB [9]. Interestingly, there has been accumulating report on patients who developed attacks of acute NB during the course of chronic progressive NB, which can be nominated as "acute on chronic" [24]. Thus, the patients recovered from attacks of acute NB by treatment with corticosteroids, whereas their manifestations of chronic progressive

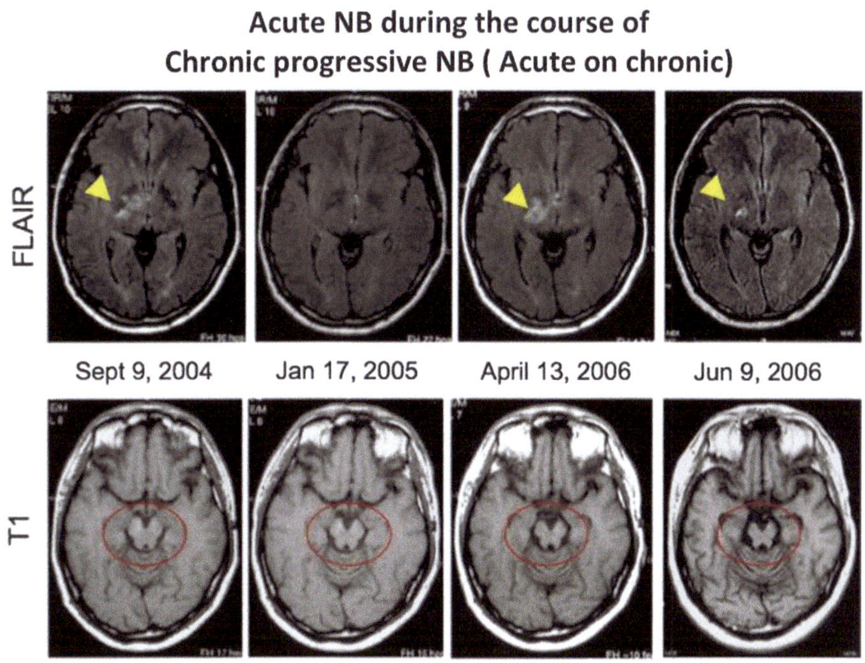

Fig. 6.3 Clinical course and changes in laboratory data of a patient who showed an attack of acute NB during the course of chronic progressive NB (From Ref.[24])

NB were not improved with continuous progression of brainstem atrophy (Fig. 6.3) [24]. These patients provide strong evidence that the pathogenesis of acute NB is different from that of chronic progressive NB [24].

6.3 Histopathology

The characteristics of histopathology of acute NB, chronic progressive NB, and NB in a long-term remission at autopsy have been delineated [25]. Thus, perivascular infiltration of mononuclear cells around small vessels (Fig. 6.4a), consisting mainly of CD45RO+ T lymphocytes and CD68+ monocytes with few CD20+ B lymphocytes, is one of the characteristic features of histopathology of the lesions in acute NB. Interestingly, most neurons were undergoing apoptosis in the inflammatory lesions with the formation of a binucleated neuron, as revealed by Tunnel staining (Fig. 6.4b) [25]. Somewhat surprisingly, the histopathological changes in chronic progressive NB were basically similar to those in acute NB. Thus, perivascular cuffing of CD45RO+ T lymphocytes and CD68+ monocytes was noted in the pons, cerebellum, medulla, internal capsule, and midbrain but less markedly compared

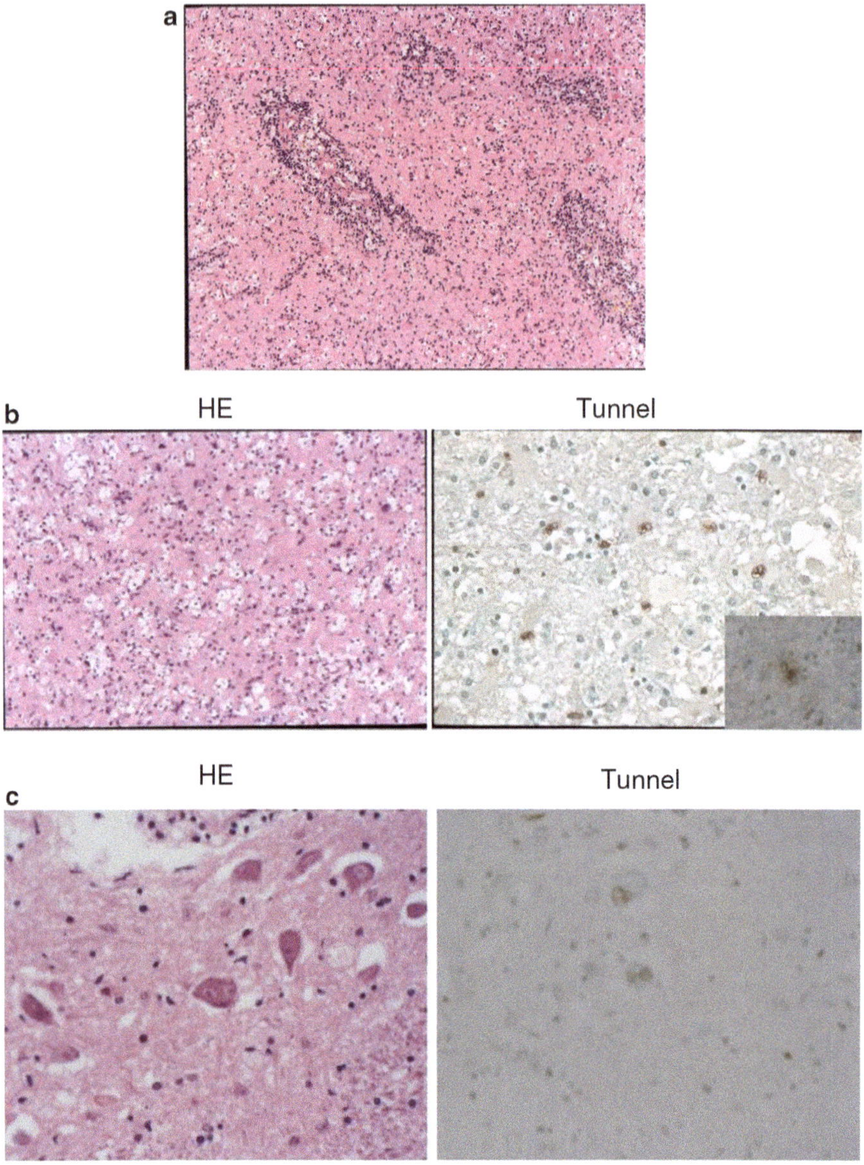

Fig. 6.4 Histopathology of lesions in the brain in acute NB and chronic progressive NB. (**a**) acute NB, HE ×25; (**b**) acute NB, HE ×25 and Tunnel ×25 (×50 in lower right); and (**c**) chronic progressive NB, HE ×25 and Tunnel ×25 (From Ref. [25])

with that in acute NB. There were also scattered foci of neurons undergoing apoptosis with a few binucleated neurons (Fig. 6.4c) [25]. On the other hand, the most prominent feature of NB in a long-term remission after the attacks of acute NB was atrophy of basal pons with cystic or moth-eaten lesions, consisting of isomorphic gliosis with viable neurons. Surprisingly, there were still scattered foci of perivascular cuffing of T lymphocytes and monocytes in NB in a long-term remission [25]. These results underscore perivascular cuffing of T lymphocytes and monocytes as the common features throughout the courses of NB irrespective of the clinical phenotypes. Since a huge amount of IL-6 is present in CSF of acute NB or chronic progressive NB, soluble factors produced by infiltrating cells, mainly IL-6, might play a critical role in the induction of apoptosis of neurons in NB.

6.4 Diagnosis

6.4.1 MRI Findings

High-intensity lesions on FLAIR images or T2-weighted images of MRI especially in brainstem-diencephalon and pontobulbar regions have been found to be frequently observed in NB [26]. Although these high-intensity lesions were most frequently seen in acute NB, they are also found in chronic progressive NB and non-NB [5]. Thus, these high-intensity lesions on MRI were detected in as many as 42.4 % of non-NB patients but as few as 60.5 % of acute NB patients [5]. Therefore, it is evident that such abnormal MRI findings are neither so frequent nor specific for acute NB, providing insufficient sensitivity and specificity for diagnosis. By contrast, brainstem atrophy was much more frequently observed in chronic progressive NB (71.4 %) than in acute NB (7.5 %) or non-NB (9.0 %), providing sufficient sensitivity and specificity for the diagnosis of chronic progressive NB and therefore can be included in the diagnostic criteria [5].

6.4.2 CSF Findings

Efficacy of CSF analysis in the diagnosis of NB has not been fully explored previously [6, 8]. Thus, in a study of a limited number of patients, CSF constituents have been shown to be altered in only around 70–80 % of patients with parenchymal NB [12]. Of note, CSF cell counts were significantly elevated in acute NB compared with non-NB and chronic progressive NB in our retrospective multicenter cohort study [5]. Although CSF cell counts were also higher in chronic progressive NB than those in non-NBD, approximately 15 % of patients with chronic progressive NB showed normal CSF cell counts [5]. As to CSF total protein or CSF glucose levels, the changes were significant but too modest to be used for differential diagnosis of acute NB or chronic progressive NB from non-NB [5].

Increasing attention has been recently paid to CSF IL-6 in NB. Thus, CSF IL-6 has been found to be elevated in patients with relapsing-remitting NB (acute NB) as well as in those with progressive NB (chronic progressive NB) [9, 27–31]. Accordingly, CSF IL-6 was shown to be elevated in acute NB as well as in chronic progressive NB, but not in non-NB in our retrospective multicenter cohort study [5]. It should be noted that CSF IL-6 was elevated only during attacks and decreased in remission phase in acute NB. By contrast, marked elevation of CSF IL-6 is sustained in chronic progressive NB in spite of modest changes in CSF cell counts and total proteins. It is therefore important to examine CSF IL-6 in remission phase of acute NB to rule out the possibility that such patients with acute NB might develop chronic progressive NB.

6.4.3 Diagnostic Criteria

In order to establish the diagnostic criteria for acute NB and chronic progressive NB, receiver operating characteristic (ROC) analysis of various parameters was performed for evaluation of suitability for inclusion in the criteria. The sensitivity and specificity of CSF cell count for diagnosis of acute NB versus non-NB were 97.4 % and 97.0 %, respectively, at the cutoff value of 6.2/mm^3 (Fig. 6.5a). However, the sensitivity of CSF cell count for diagnosis of chronic progressive NB against non-NB was only 68.6 % at the cutoff value of 6.0/mm^3 [5].

It should be noted that chronic progressive NB often develops following the episodes of acute NB [8, 9]. It is therefore important to determine whether patients of the recovery phase of acute NB might develop chronic progressive NB. ROC analysis was thus carried out between patients with chronic progressive NB and those who did not develop chronic progressive NB during recovery phase of acute NB. The results disclosed that the sensitivity and specificity of CSF IL-6 for diagnosis of chronic progressive NB were 92.0 % and 94.7 %, respectively, at the cutoff value of 16.55 pg/ml (Fig. 6.5b) [5].

These results confirm that CSF IL-6 was a useful marker for diagnosis of chronic progressive NB in BD patients who showed neurological manifestations

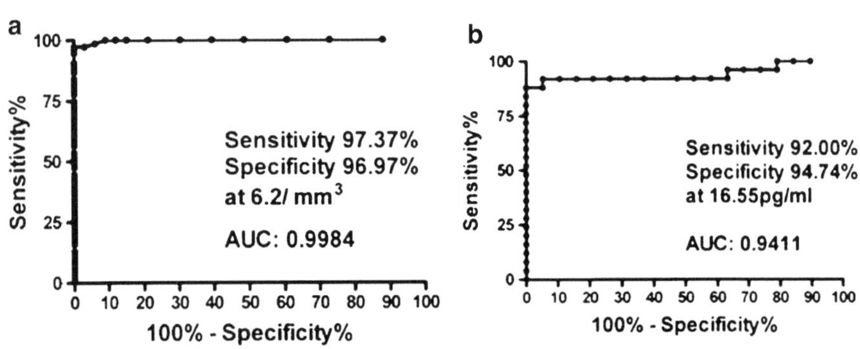

Fig. 6.5 Receiver operating characteristic (ROC) analysis of CSF cell count and CSF IL-6 for differential diagnosis of NB. (**a**) ROC analysis of CSF cell count for differential diagnosis of acute NBD from non-NBD. Area under the curve (AUC). (**b**) ROC analysis of CSF IL-6 for diagnosis of CP NB versus acute NB in recovery phase (Modified from Ref. [5])

Table 6.2 Proposed preliminary diagnostic criteria for classification of NB

Acute NB
1. Fulfilling the ISD criteria for BS
2. Acute or subacute onset of neurological symptoms, including headache, fever with or without any focal signs
3. Increase in CSF cell number over 6.2/mm^3
*The diagnosis of acute NB requires all the above items 1–3
Exclusion: infections of the central nervous system
Note: There is a subtype associated with cyclosporine A (CyA)
Chronic progressive NB
1. Fulfilling the ISD criteria for BS
2. Insidious onset of neuropsychiatric symptoms, including dementia/neurobehavior changes, ataxia, dysarthria with or without other manifestations
3. Presence of one of the following:
(a) Increase in CSF IL-6 over 16.55 pg/ml on 2 different occasions with intervals of at least 2 weeks
(b) Increase in CSF IL-6 over 16.55 pg/ml and the presence of brainstem atrophy on MRI
*The diagnosis of chronic progressive NB requires all the above items 1–3

Modified from Ref. [5]

of insidious onset. CSF cell count was a sensitive and reliable marker only for diagnosis of acute NB in BD patients who showed neurological manifestations of acute or subacute onset. It should be underscored that CSF IL-6 and cell count have been found to be elevated in CNS infections. Therefore, it is mandatory to rule out CNS infections, especially in acute NB. Moreover, it should be noted that a fraction of BD patients treated with CyA develop acute neurological events that could not be discriminated with acute NB [5]. It makes sense that such neurological manifestations should be considered acute NB as well, since there were no significant changes in various features and parameters between CyA-associated events and CyA-unassociated events [5]. As shown in Table 6.2, the diagnostic criteria for acute NB and chronic progressive NB were proposed, based on these findings [5].

6.5 Treatment

It is important to recognize that treatment of NB is different depending on its presentation: acute NB and chronic progressive NB. As to acute NB, treatment of acute phase manifestations as well as prevention of recurrent attacks should be considered separately [7].

6.5.1 Acute NB

6.5.1.1 Acute Phase Manifestations

Corticosteroids are the golden standards to treat active phase in acute NB, but their effects are short-lived and they do not prevent recurrence of attacks [12]. Consistently, more than 80 % of the patients with acute NB were treated with corticosteroid during the acute attacks in our retrospective multicenter cohort [5]. The patients are usually given oral prednisolone (1 mg/kg for up to 4 weeks or until improvement is observed) with or without high-dose intravenous methylprednisolone (1 g/day) for 3–7 days [32]. After the attacks subside by treatment, the doses of corticosteroids should be decreased gradually over 2–3 months in order to prevent early relapses [32]. Although intravenous methylprednisolone pulse therapy has been suggested to result in earlier improvement, there has been no controlled study to demonstrate its efficacy.

In addition to corticosteroids, the efficacy of interferon alpha (IFN-α2a) has been suggested in the treatment of the active phase manifestations of acute NB as well as ocular manifestations [33]. Further controlled study is required to confirm this point.

Recent clinical trials have demonstrated that infliximab is effective in preventing the recurrence of ocular attacks and has beneficial effects for the visual prognosis of patients with refractory uveoretinitis [34, 35]. Several reports have also suggested the efficacy of infliximab for acute NB [28, 36]. Thus, an improvement in symptoms was noticed within 24 h after receiving the first infusion and remained stable throughout the course with a complete resolution of signal abnormalities on brain MRI [36]. A similar patient with brainstem lesions in acute NB who responded well to infliximab was reported [28].

On the other hand, it should be underscored that the neurological involvement of acute NB occasionally subsides spontaneously [37]. Taken together, it is recommended that the use of corticosteroids, IFN-α2a, and infliximab should be considered depending on the severity and the course of attacks of acute NB based on careful evaluation, since spontaneous remission might be possible.

6.5.1.2 Prevention of Relapse of Acute NB

A variety of drugs, including colchicine, azathioprine, CyA, cyclophosphamide, MTX, chlorambucil, and immunomodulatory agents such as IFN-α, pentoxyphilline, and thalidomide, have been anecdotally used for prevention of the occurrence of the systemic manifestations of BD, but none of these agents have been demonstrated to be effective in preventing the attacks of acute NB in a controlled study [7, 11, 12]. CyA has been reported to result in neurotoxicity or to accelerate the development of CNS symptoms, and therefore its use in NB is not recommended [7, 11, 21]. Rather, accumulating studies have suggested that CyA induces acute NB [21]. Thus, there were no significant differences in demographic features, clinical symptoms, MRI findings, and the need for and responses to corticosteroid therapy including pulse therapy between patients with CyA-related acute NB and CyA-unrelated acute NB [5]. It is therefore recommended that CyA should not be used in patients with preceding history of acute NB whether the previous attacks were associated with the use of CyA or not.

6.5.2 Chronic Progressive NB

Immunosuppressive drugs, such as azathioprine, and oral or intravenous cyclophosphamide along with high-dose corticosteroid have been usually administered in chronic progressive NB; however, a number of miserable courses under such treatment regimens have clearly demonstrated their ineffectiveness [7–9]. Thus, it should be emphasized that high doses of corticosteroid are not at all effective in chronic progressive NB [9]. Thus, the patients usually show exacerbation along with continuing marked elevation of CSF IL-6 even when higher doses of corticosteroid are used [9]. Neither cyclophosphamide, regardless of oral or intravenous administration, nor azathioprine has been shown to prevent progression [9].

We happened to experience a patient with chronic progressive NB, who dramatically responded to low-dose weekly MTX with dramatic decrease in CSF IL-6 activity. The following open trial with 6 patients with chronic progressive NB revealed that the neuropsychological manifestations as well as the findings on MRI scans and intelligence quotients were not significantly worsened during the trial with MTX [23]. As to toxicity of MTX, 3 patients presented with mild liver dysfunction, which returned to normal by decreasing the dose of MTX. Further studies of low-dose weekly MTX for a longer period (4 years) confirmed its beneficial effects in chronic progressive NB [38]. Thus, these results indicate that low-dose weekly MTX is tolerable and beneficial in the treatment of patients with chronic progressive NB, since it prevented the progression of the neuropsychiatric manifestations by significantly decreasing CSF IL-6.

It should be emphasized, however, there are still a fraction of patients with chronic progressive NB, who did not adequately respond to MTX [38]. Notably, it has been reported that infliximab was effective for the treatment of long-standing recalcitrant chronic progressive NB [39, 40]. We also explored the efficacy of infliximab in 5 patients with chronic progressive NB refractory to MTX. These patients were given intravenous infusion of infliximab (5 mg/kg at weeks 0, 2, 6, and 14) along with MTX (10–17.5 mg/week) and prednisolone (<10 mg/day). In all the 5 patients, CSF IL-6 were markedly decreased by 1/2–1/37 on the next day of the 1st infusion of infliximab and stayed below 20 pg/ml before the last infusion at 14 weeks. By contrast, CSF TNF-α levels were not significantly changed at any time point [41]. At 24 weeks from the initial infusion, none of the 5 patients showed neurological exacerbation and 3 patients significantly improved. Accordingly, MRI scans showed no progression of the atrophy in the midbrain, pons, and medulla [41]. Adverse events occurred in 2 of the 5 patients, including transient headache in one patient and subclinical pneumocystis pneumonia in the other patient [41]. Thus, it was suggested that infliximab might have a beneficial effect in the treatment of chronic progressive NB by reducing CSF IL-6 levels but not TNF-α. Moreover, the rapid decrease in CSF IL-6 after the infusion indicates the direct interaction of infliximab with inflammatory cells producing IL-6 [41, 42].

It should be noted that etanercept was effective in suppressing most of the mucocutaneous manifestations in BD [43]. Therefore, clinical studies to explore the efficacy of etanercept in the treatment of chronic progressive NB would be worthwhile. Persistent marked elevation of CSF IL-6 is a hallmark of chronic progress NB. Therefore, treatment with tocilizumab, an anti-IL-6 receptor monoclonal antibody, might also have beneficial effects. In fact, tocilizumab has been shown to be effective in a patient with progressive NB with high CSF IL-6 activities, who did not adequately respond to infliximab [44]. A further clinical trial of tocilizumab is therefore warranted.

6.6 Conclusion

A variety neurological and neuropsychological manifestations can be presented due to CVT or parenchymal involvement in BD. The latter is called as NB, consisting of acute NB and chronic progressive NB. Since treatment regimens are totally different, correct diagnosis of both types of NB is quite important. Diagnostic criteria for both types of NB have been now established. As for treatment, administration of corticosteroid should be considered depending on the severity of the attack in acute NB. For prevention of the relapse of attacks of acute NB, colchicine and tapering corticosteroid are anecdotally used. On the other hand, one should realize that corticosteroids and cyclophosphamide are not effective at all in chronic progressive NB. Low-dose weekly MTX is an anchor drug for chronic progressive NB and infliximab has been also shown to be effective in recalcitrant cases, as is in the case with rheumatoid arthritis. Furthermore, tocilizumab appears to be promising.

References

1. Hirohata S, Kikuchi H. Behçet's disease. Arthritis Res Ther. 2003;5:139–46.
2. Jennette JC, Falk RJ, Bacon PA, Basu N, Cid MC, et al. 2012 revised International Chapel Hill Consensus Conference Nomenclature of Vasculitides. Arthritis Rheum. 2013;65:1–11.
3. Serdaroglu P. Behçet's disease and the nervous system. J Neurol. 1998;245:197–205.
4. Ideguchi H, Suda A, Takeno M, Kirino Y, Ihata A, et al. Neurological manifestations of Behçet's disease in Japan: a study of 54 patients. J Neurol. 2010;257:1012–20.
5. Hirohata S, Kikuchi H, Sawada T, Nagafuchi H, Kuwana M, et al. Clinical characteristics of neuro-Behcet's disease in Japan: a multicenter retrospective analysis. Mod Rheumatol. 2012;22:405–13.
6. Kidd D, Steuer A, Denman AM, Rudge P. Neurological complications in Behçet's syndrome. Brain. 1999;122:2183–94.

7. Siva A, Altintas A, Saip S. Behçet's syndrome and the nervous system. Curr Opin Neurol. 2004;17:347–57.
8. Akman-Demir G, Serdaroglu P, Tasci B, The Neuro-Behçet Study Group. Clinical patterns of neurological involvement in Behçet's disease: evaluation of 200 patients. Brain. 1999;122:2171–82.
9. Hirohata S, Isshi K, Oguchi H, Ohse T, Haraoka H, Takeuchi A, Hashikmoto T. Cerebrospinal fluid interleukin-6 in progressive Neuro-Behcet's syndrome. Clin Immunol Immunopathol. 1997;82:12–7.
10. Hirohata S. Potential new therapeutic options for involvement of central nervous system in Behçet's disease (Neuro- Behçet's syndrome). Curr Rheumatol Rev. 2007;3:297–303.
11. Siva A, Hirohata S. Behçet's syndrome and the nervous. In: Yazici Y, Yazici H, editors. Behçet's syndrome. New York: Springer; 2010. p. 95–113.
12. Al-Araji A, Kidd D. Neuro-Behçet's disease: epidemiology, clinical characteristics, and management. Lancet Neurol. 2009;8:192–204.
13. Saadoun D, Wechsler B, Resche-Rigon M, et al. Cerebral venous thrombosis in Behçet's disease. Arthritis Rheum. 2009;61:518–26.
14. Wechsler B, Vidailhet M, Bousser MG, et al. Cerebral venous sinus thrombosis in Behçet's disease: long term follow-up of 25 cases. Neurology. 1992;42:614–8.
15. Siva A, Kantarci OH, Saip S, et al. Behçet's disease: diagnostic and prognostic aspects of neurological involvement. J Neurol. 2001;248:95–103.
16. Tunc R, Saib S, Siva A, Yazici H. Cerebral venous thrombosis is associated with major vessel disease in Behcet's syndrome. Ann Rheum Dis. 2004;63:1693–4.
17. Houman MH, Hamzaoui-B'Chir S, Ben Ghorbel I, et al. Neurologic manifestations of Behcet's disease: analysis of a series of 27 patients. Rev Med Interne. 2002;23:592–606.
18. Ideguchi H, Suda A, Takeno M, Ueda A, Ohno S, et al. Characteristics of vascular involvement in Behçet's disease in Japan: a retrospective cohort study. Clin Exp Rheumatol. 2011;29(4 Suppl 67):S47–53.
19. Saip S, Siva A, Altintas A, Kiyat A, Seyahi E, Hamuryudan V, Yazici H. Headache in Behçet's syndrome. Headache. 2005;45:911–9.
20. Lo Monaco A, La Corte R, Caniatti L, Borrelli M, Trotta F. Neurological involvement in North Italian patients with Behçet disease. Rheumatol Int. 2006;26:1113–9.
21. Kotake S, Higashi K, Yoshikawa K, Sasamoto Y, Okamoto T, Matsuda H. Central nervous system symptoms in patients with Behçet disease receiving cyclosporine therapy. Ophthalmology. 1999;106:586–9.
22. Aramaki K, Kikuchi H, Hirohata S. HLA-B51 and cigarette smoking as risk factors for chronic progressive neurological manifestations in Behcet's disease. Mod Rheumatol. 2007;17:81–2.
23. Hirohata S, Suda H, Hashimoto T. Low-dose weekly methotrexate for progressive neuropsychiatric manifestations in Behçet's disease. J Neurol Sci. 1998;159:181–5.
24. Matsui T, Ishida T, Tono T, Yoshida T, Sato S-I, et al. An attack of acute neuro-Behçet's disease during the course of chronic progressive neuro-Behçet's disease: report of two cases. Mod Rheumatol. 2010;20:621–6.
25. Hirohata S. Histopathology of central nervous system lesions in Behçet's disease. J Neurol Sci. 2008;267:41–7.
26. Koçer N, Islak C, Siva A, Saip S, Akman C, Kantarci O, et al. CNS involvement in neuro-Behçet's syndrome: an MR study. Am J Neuroradiol. 1999;20:1015–24.
27. Hirohata S, Takeuchi A, Miyamoto T. Elevated levels of interleukin 6 in cerebrospinal fluid from patients with Neuro-Behçet's syndrome. In: O'Duffy JD, Kokmen E, editors. Behçet's disease. New York: Marcel Dekker; 1991. p. 369–76.
28. Fujikawa K, Aratake K, Kawakami A, Aramaki T, Iwanaga N, Izumi Y, et al. Successful treatment of refractory neuro-Behcet's disease with infliximab: a case report to show its efficacy by magnetic resonance imaging, transcranial magnetic stimulation and cytokine profile. Ann Rheum Dis. 2007;66:136–7.
29. Akman-Demir G, Tüzün E, Içöz S, Yeşilot N, Yentür SP, Kürtüncü M, et al. Interleukin-6 in neuro-Behçet's disease: association with disease subsets and long-term outcome. Cytokine. 2008;44:373–6.

30. Haghighi AB, Ittehadi H, Nikseresht AR, Rahmati J, Poorjahromi SG, Pourabbas B, et al. CSF levels of cytokines in neuro-Behçet's disease. Clin Neurol Neurosurg. 2009;111:507–10.
31. Hirohata S, Kikuchi H. Changes in biomarkers focused on differences in disease course or treatment in patients with Neuro-Behçet's disease. Intern Med. 2012;51:3359–65.
32. Siva A, Fresko I. Behçet's disease. Curr Treat Options Neurol. 2000;2:435–48.
33. Nichols JC, Ince A, Akduman L, Mann ES. Interferon-alpha 2a treatment of neuro-Behçet disease. J Neuroophthalmol. 2001;21:109–11.
34. Ohno S, Nakamura S, Hori S, Shimakawa M, Kawashima H, Mochizuki M, Sugita S, Ueno S, Yoshizaki K, Inaba G. Efficacy, safety, and pharmacokinetics of multiple administration of infliximab in Behçet's disease with refractory uveoretinitis. J Rheumatol. 2004;31:1362–8.
35. Tugal-Tutkun I, Mudun A, Urgancioglu M, Kamali S, Kasapoglu E, Inanc M, Gul A. Efficacy of infliximab in the treatment of uveitis that is resistant to treatment with the combination of azathioprine, cyclosporine, and corticosteroids in Behçet's disease: an open-label trial. Arthritis Rheum. 2005;52:2478–84.
36. Licata G, Pinto A, Tuttolomondo A, Banco A, Ciccia F, Ferrante A, Triolo G. Anti-tumour necrosis factor alpha monoclonal antibody therapy for recalcitrant cerebral vasculitis in a patient with Behçet's syndrome. Ann Rheum Dis. 2003;62:280–1.
37. Hirohata S, Kamoshita H, Taketani T. Spontaneous remission of meningoencephalitis in Behçet's disease. J Rheumatol. 1989;16:1283–4.
38. Kikuchi H, Aramaki K, Hirohata S. Low dose MTX for progressive neuro- Behçet's disease. A follow-up study for 4 years. Adv Exp Med Biol. 2003;528:575–8.
39. Sarwar H, McGrath Jr H, Espinoza LR. Successful treatment of long-standing neuro-Behcet's disease with infliximab. J Rheumatol. 2005;32:181–3.
40. Piptone N, Olivieri I, Padula A, D'angelo S, Nigro A, et al. Infliximab for the treatment of neuro-Behçet's disease: a case series and review of the literature. Arthritis Rheum. 2008;59:285–90.
41. Kikuchi H, Aramaki K, Hirohata S. Effect of infliximab in progressive Neuro-Behcet's syndrome. J Neurol Sci. 2008;272:99–105.
42. Mitoma H, Horiuchi T, Tsukamoto H, Tamimoto Y, Kimoto Y, Uchino A, To K, Harashima S, Hatta N, Harada M. Mechanisms for cytotoxic effects of anti-tumor necrosis factor agents on transmembrane tumor necrosis factor alpha-expressing cells: comparison among infliximab, etanercept, and adalimumab. Arthritis Rheum. 2008;58:1248–57.
43. Melikoglu M, Fresko I, Mat C, Ozyazgan Y, Gogus F, Yurdakul S, Hamuryudan V, Yazici H. Short-term trial of etanercept in Behçet's disease: a double blind, placebo controlled study. J Rheumatol. 2005;32:98–105.
44. Urbaniak P, Hasler P, Kretzschmar S. Refractory neuro-Behçet treated by tocilizumab: a case report. Clin Exp Rheumatol. 2012; 3(Suppl 72):S73–5.

Chapter 7
Gastrointestinal Involvement

Masakazu Nagahori

Abstract The prevalence of gastrointestinal involvement varies greatly between different areas of the world for unknown reasons. Although it is considered to be relatively uncommon complications, it could pose a significant impact on the patient's quality of life due to repeated hospitalizations and even surgeries. Because well-designed therapeutic trials are quite limited, current medical management is mostly empirical and unsatisfactory from both efficacy and safety standpoints. The advent of anti-TNF-α agents could meet the unmet needs for the patients and remarkably change our current management, setting the therapeutic goal from symptomatic improvement to improved prognosis by achieving mucosal healing. Increasing our knowledge about the prognosis is also expected to be helpful in customizing the therapeutic strategy for each patient.

Keywords Volcano-type ulcer • Disease activity index for intestinal Behçet's disease (DAIBD) • Anti-TNF therapy

7.1 Introduction

Development of new imaging modalities, especially endoscopic examinations, has allowed us to investigate various gastrointestinal (GI) diseases such as inflammatory bowel diseases, including GI involvement of Behçet's disease. However, as its another name as "Silk Road disease" shows, its GI involvement has not been satisfactorily investigated in countries such as in North America and Europe where advanced medical technologies are available for the investigation. Recent investigations and reports from East Asian countries such as Japan and Korea have enabled us to understand the pathophysiology and prognosis of the

M. Nagahori (✉)
Department of Gastroenterology and Hepatology,
Tokyo Medical and Dental University, Tokyo, Japan
e-mail: nagahori.gast@tmd.ac.jp

Y. Ishigatsubo (ed.), *Behçet's Disease*,
DOI 10.1007/978-4-431-54487-6_7

intestinal disease. The advent of effect treatments such as anti-TNF-α agents will also give our patients and us an opportunity for improvement of the patients' symptoms and quality of life.

In this chapter, our latest knowledge about the GI involvement will be described, being focused upon the prognosis and emerging treatments.

7.2 Prevalence of GI Manifestations

The epidemiology of GI involvement in Behçet's disease (BD) varies substantially among the different parts of the world, which is well manifested by the widely different prevalences of GI manifestations (Table 7.1) [1]. They are seen in as high as 16 % in Japan and only 2.8 % in Turkey. The reason of such wide variability is unknown. Childhood-onset BD patients who develop symptoms at age 16 or before are suggested to have different expressions and severity of manifestations, where GI symptoms and intestinal ulcers might be more common than in adult-onset BD patients [2, 3].

Table 7.1 Distribution of gastrointestinal manifestations of BD in the world

Area	Number of cases	Prevalence (%)
Iran	5,059	7.6
Japan	3,316	16
China	1,996	8.8
Korea	1,527	7.3
Germany	590	12
Turkey	2,147	2.8
Morocco	1,034	11
UK	419	7
Saudi Arabia	119	4
Iraq	58	3.3
Jordan	150	20
Lebanon	100	10
Egypt	274	10
Algeria	58	5
Russia	35	37
Italy	155	34
France	73	18
USA	164	8
Spain	38	5

7.3 Esophageal Lesions

Symptomatic esophageal involvement is very uncommon [4]. It usually involves the middle part of the esophagus. Common symptoms are substernal pain and dysphagia. However, hematemesis is relatively uncommon. Endoscopic findings show erosions, aphthous, linear, or perforating ulcers, and occasional diffuse esophagitis. Possible complications are perforation, dissection, penetration, fistula, and stenosis. Histological findings are often nonspecific inflammation, and vasculitis is rare. Surveillance endoscopy is not recommended in asymptomatic patients because nonspecific esophageal findings found in such patients are not severe enough to be associated with complications [5].

7.4 Gastric and Duodenal Lesions

The stomach is the least frequently involved part in GI tract, although as high as 43 % of BD patients were reported to have gastric or duodenal ulcers from Taiwan [6]. Case reports showed pyloric stenosis due to edematous hypertrophy of the pyloric ring or a Dieulafoy's ulcer [7–9]. Prospective endoscopic evaluation in asymptomatic patients might show frequent nonspecific abnormalities such as hiatal hernia, gastritis, and gastric and duodenal ulceration [10]. They also reported no difference of *Helicobacter pylori* prevalence, compared to control group. On the other hand, in BD patients who have upper GI symptoms, lesions found by endoscopic examination are most likely to be nonspecific gastritis or duodenitis [11, 12].

7.5 Intestinal Lesions

Intestinal mucosal lesions are the most common GI involvement and are characterized by solitary or multiple deep ulcers most typically in the ileocecal region and colon (Fig. 7.1). Presenting symptoms vary from right lower quadrant abdominal pain, diarrhea, or hematochezia to acute abdomen due to penetration or perforation. Macroscopic characterization of colonic ulcers is helpful in predicting the clinical course of each patient [13]. The volcano-type ones had a poor response to medical treatment and required surgery more frequently and recurred more often than geographic-type and aphthous-type ulcers. Differential diagnosis from Crohn's disease (CD) is occasionally difficult because both typically involve the ileocecal area and show discrete and discontinuous ulcers. Pathological examinations of biopsy specimen usually show a vasculitis of the small veins but no granulomas. The colonoscopic characterizations of ulcers are helpful in differentiating between intestinal BD and CD, being round or oval with a punched-out appearance in the former and longitudinal in the latter. Lee et al. made up a simple decision tree to differentiate between intestinal BD and CD by classification and regression analysis (Fig. 7.2) [14]. The International Study Group criteria for BD

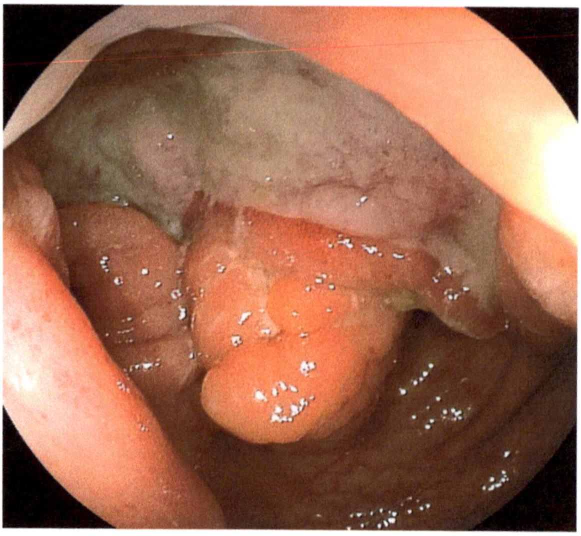

Fig. 7.1 Colonoscopic image of the solitary volcano-type ulcer in the ileocecal area in a patient with BD

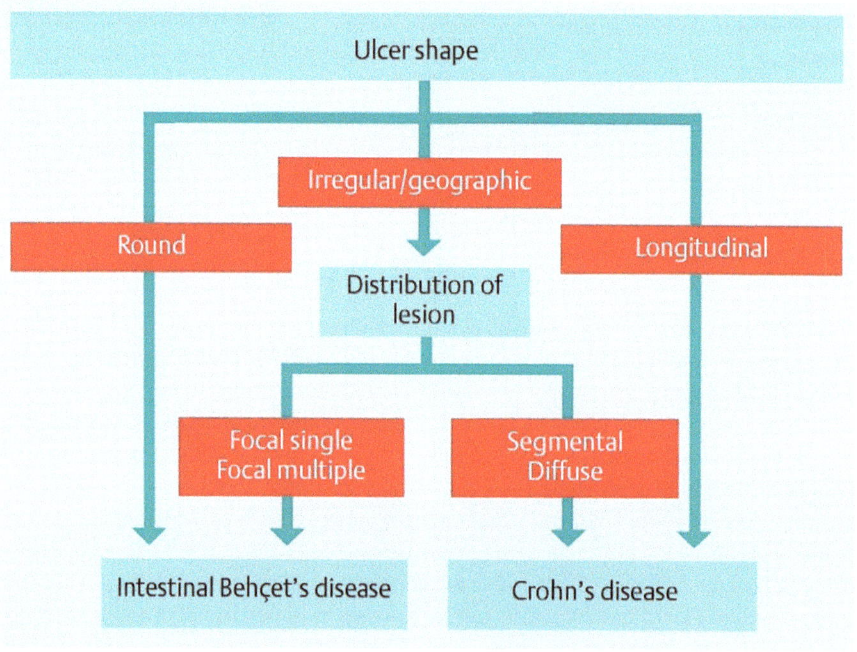

Fig. 7.2 The decision tree to differentiate between intestinal Behçet's disease and Crohn's disease

was also evaluated about its accuracy in differentiating BD from familial Mediterranean fever and inflammatory bowel disease such as ulcerative colitis and Crohn's disease and was reported to have high sensitivity and specificity [15]. However, in a daily practice, it is not uncommon to see a patient in whom differential diagnosis between these two is impossible. In addition to the role in differential diagnosis, microscopic examination in the ileum might reveal abnormal histologies even in BD patients without macroscopic abnormalities in ileum and colon [16].

Cross-sectional imaging, such as computed tomography (CT) and magnetic resonance imaging (MRI), provides valuable information which enables us to understand the transmural pathophysiology beyond mucosal inflammation. CT scan shows concentric or uneven bowel wall thickening with remarkable contrast enhancement. It could also reveal complications such as bowel perforation with or without perforation and penetration. CT scanning is also valuable in differentiating BD from appendicitis when the patient presents with acute right lower quadrant pain with local peritonitis. MRI also reveals wall thickening with contrast enhancement. In some patients, extraintestinal findings such as mesenteric infiltration around the involved bowel can be evaluated as well [17].

Video capsule endoscopy (VCE) is widely used for suspected small bowel diseases. It should be considered for identifying small bowel lesions in patients with established diagnosis of BD who have GI symptoms, particularly when conventional investigations are not able to pinpoint lesions to account for the symptoms [18, 19]. Interestingly enough, Neves et al. reported that jejunal lesions were found in 80 %(8/10) of the patients evaluated by VCE, which give us an opportunity to reconsider the widely known knowledge that ileocecal area is the most affected location in GI tract [19].

Because the disease activity of intestinal disease considerably fluctuates over time and even spontaneous resolution is not uncommon, there has been no disease activity index such as those in Crohn's disease and ulcerative colitis available for intestinal BD until recently. Disease activity index for intestinal Behçet's disease (DAIBD) is an instrument for the numerical measurement of disease activity in patients with intestinal BD, which is a simple 8-point index, easily administered in an office setting (Table 7.2) [20]. However, the correlation between DAIBD and endoscopic severity was reported to be weak ($r=0.434$) [21].

7.6 GI Vascular Lesions

Abdominal vasculitis more often affects small veins and venules than arteries and arterioles. Pathological examination shows intense inflammation around the vasa vasorum, which results in destruction of the media and fibrous thickening of the intima and adventitia [22]. Although thrombosis and aneurysm of the large arteries in the abdomen is considered to be quite uncommon, a case who developed intestinal infarction due to superior mesenteric artery thrombosis was reported [23]. Another case report described a case with intestinal perforation secondary to aneurysmal occlusion of superior mesenteric artery [24].

Table 7.2 Disease activity index for intestinal Behçet's disease

Items	Score
General well-being for 1 week	
Well	0
Fair	10
Poor	20
Very poor	30
Terrible	40
Fever	
<38 °C	0
≥38 °C	10
Extraintestinal manifestations[a]	5 per item
Abdominal pain in 1 week	
None	0
Mild	20
Moderate	40
Severe	80
Abdominal mass	
None	0
Palpable mass	10
Abdominal tenderness	
None	0
Mildly tender	10
Moderately or severely tender	20
Intestinal complications[b]	10 per item
No. of liquid stools in 1 week	
0	0
1–7	10
8–21	20
22–35	30
≥36	40

[a]Score 5 for oral ulcer, genital ulcer, eye lesion, skin lesion, or arthralgia; score 15 for vascular involvement or central nervous system involvement

[b]Fistula, perforation, abscess, or intestinal obstruction

7.7 Treatment

Although evidence-based treatment is quite limited in managing gastrointestinal involvement in BD, medical therapies such as sulfasalazine, corticosteroids, azathioprine, and anti-TNF antagonists are recommended by EULAR except for patients in surgical emergencies [25].

Treatment of esophageal lesions usually comprises corticosteroids and no improvement used to be expected by proton pump inhibitors. Systemic anti-inflammatory effect of mesalazine was suggested in a case report to be effective for esophageal ulcers in BD

[26]. Although optimal management is still unknown, a Korean center experience showed successful treatment in most patients by medical therapies that included mesalazine, proton pump inhibitors, and/or colchicines [27].

Gastric and duodenal lesions may be difficult to be treated by medical therapies with antiulcer medications. Although the role of immunosuppressive medications is unknown, good response to corticosteroid was reported from Taiwan in patients with gastric and duodenal ulcers [6]. Although the role of *Helicobacter pylori* is unknown in gastric and duodenal lesions in BD, the eradication therapy might be considered, expecting the improvement of oral and genital ulcers [28].

Although good evidence is still limited about the efficacy of 5-ASA agents for the intestinal disease, they are recommended as the first-line therapy for mild to moderate disease because of the favorable safety profile, except for occasional allergic reactions [29]. Optimal doses of mesalazine and sulfasalazine are 2.25–3 g/day and 3–4 g/day, respectively. When remission is obtained, they can be continued as maintenance therapy. However, relapse is common during the long-term treatment. Cumulative relapse rate was reported to be 8.1 %, 22.6 %, 31.2 %, and 46.7 % at 1, 3, 5, and 10 years after remission induced by 5-ASA or sulfasalazine [30], respectively. They also reported a younger age at diagnosis (<35 years), higher C-reactive protein level (≥1.5 mg/dL), and a higher DAIBD (≥60) were factors associated with relapse during the maintenance therapy.

Corticosteroid is used for patients who do not respond to 5-ASA and those with severe symptoms such as abdominal pain and bleeding. Induction dose of corticosteroids is 0.5–1 mg/kg per day of prednisolone for 1–2 weeks. Once improvement is observed, it should be tapered and discontinued if possible because its role as maintenance therapy is unknown both from efficacy and safety perspectives.

Although colchicine is effective for cutaneous and articular manifestations, it is not widely used in intestinal disease because of its uncertain efficacy and its GI side effects such as diarrhea and abdominal pain.

Thioprines such as azathioprine and 6-mercaptutopurine should be tried in patients who are corticosteroid dependent or corticosteroid resistant. The efficacy of thioprines as maintenance therapy for patients with medically or surgically induced remission was reported [31]. The cumulative relapse rate was 5.8 %, 28.7 %, 43.7 %, and 51.7 % at 1, 2, 3, and 5 years after remission induction, respectively. Independent predictors for relapse were younger age at diagnosis (<25 years) and lower hemoglobin level (<11 g/dL). Also, Choi et al. reported that reoperation was less likely in patients who were treated with azathioprine (7 vs. 25 % at 2 years, 25 vs. 47 % at 5 years; $p=0.035$) [32]. Consequently, postoperative use of thioprines might be considered to aim for preventing postoperative recurrence and reoperation especially for patients who are at higher risk of recurrence. Although the data is quite limited, another immunosuppressant, methotrexate could also be considered especially in those who are intolerable to thioprines. Its efficacy as combination therapy with infliximab was also reported in a case report [33].

Blocking tumor necrotic factor (TNF)-α has been gaining a great deal of attention as a promising therapeutic approach for patients with intestinal BD as well as for those with inflammatory bowel diseases. Several case reports and series have reported that infliximab, a chimeric monoclonal antibody against TNF-α, is effective for inducing and maintaining remission [34–39]. Recently, a Korean group reported efficacy and tolerability of infliximab by evaluating 28 refractory intestinal BD cases [40]. Not only did they reported response rate of 64.3 % and 50.0 % at week 4 and week 30, respectively, but they also identified five independent prognostic factors of sustained response as older age (>40 years) at diagnosis, female gender, longer disease duration (≥5 years), concomitant immunosuppressant use, and clinical remission at week 4. The role of adalimumab, a fully human anti-TNF-α monoclonal antibody, in managing intestinal disease in BD is reported only as a case report [41]. However, because its efficacy was shown in an open-label clinical trial in Japan (un-published), it was approved to be used for intestinal BD in Japan.

Because of its anti-inflammatory and immunomodulatory properties and several reports to suggest its efficacy in a variety of conditions, thalidomide, a cyclic derivative of glutamic acid, was evaluated in steroid-dependent juvenile-onset intestinal BD patients. The case series suggested its efficacy and tolerability, where 2 mg/kg/day was administered as an initial dosage. However, its use should be extremely cautious in patients of reproductive age [42].

Nutritional support, especially that by enteral nutrition, is recommended as primary therapy by the Japanese consensus statements, which were mostly decided by the expert opinions [5].

Surgical resection is indicated for patients that do not respond to medical therapy or those with intestinal complications such as stricture/obstruction, fistula/perforation/abscesses, and massive bleeding. Although there has been a controversy about the length of resection between wide and minimal surgical margin, a retrospective report showed that length of ileal resection and whether hemicolectomy was performed were not associated with recurrence or reoperation rate [32]. Intraoperative endoscopy might be considered during the operation because of its possible contribution to decrease the risk of postoperative recurrence [43].

Topical administration of absolute ethanol spray was suggested to be effective for postoperative recurrent ulcer by the experience in four such patients [44].

7.8 Prognosis

The prognosis of intestinal disease is quite variable among patients, and it is difficult to predict the natural course of each patient. However, complete remission of the intestinal lesions was reported in 38 % of patients after 8 weeks of medical therapies [32]. Also, according to the retrospective cohort study by Jung et al., most patients went into remission or had a mild clinical activity [45]. They also identified five different clinical course patterns (Fig. 7.3). Initial presentation with high DAIBD was independently associated with a severe clinical course. In addition, patients who are diagnosed in younger age before 40 years of age may have worse prognosis with higher probabilities of operation, hospital admission, and corticosteroid treatment [46].

About the postoperative recurrence, Choi et al. reported that cumulative recurrence rates were 28 %, 49 %, and 75 % at 1,2, and 5 years [32], respectively. Because the recurrence can usually be observed around the anastomotic site, surveillance colonoscopy might be considered especially in patients who are at risk of recurrence. Previous

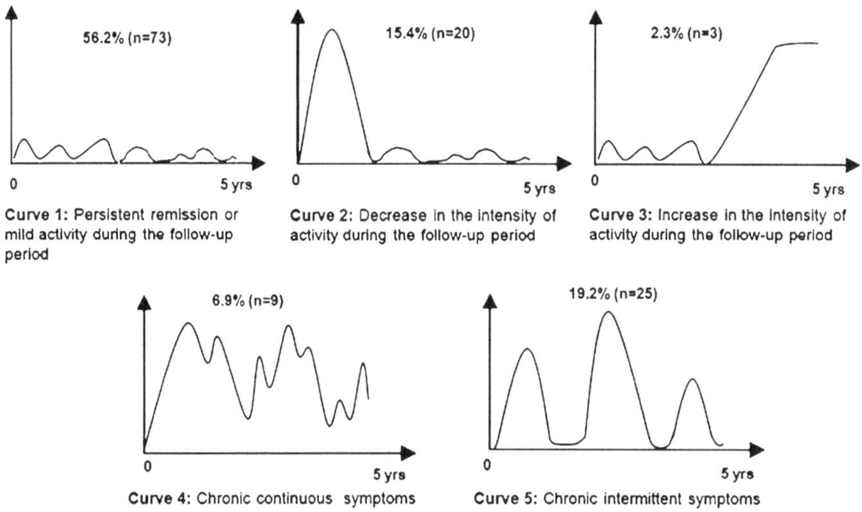

Fig. 7.3 Five different curves reflecting the clinical courses observed during the first 5-year follow-up period

surgery for fistula or perforation was reported to be a poor prognostic factor associated with postoperative endoscopic recurrence [32]. Another group identified volcano-shaped ulcers, higher C-reactive protein (CRP) levels (≥4.4 mg/dL), and the presence of intestinal perforations detected by pathology as independent predictive factors for recurrence in a multivariate analysis [47]. Likewise, reoperation is common among postoperative patients during long-term follow-up.

The role of mucosal healing as a prognostic factor is not fully evaluated among intestinal BD patients unlike IBD patients. In a retrospective analysis, patients who achieved a complete remission after 8 weeks of medical treatment were less likely to require an operation than those who did not [32]. Along with the introduction of potent medical therapies such as anti-TNF agents, mucosal healing will likely to become an achievable therapeutic goal in intestinal BD patients to maximize their prognosis.

7.9 Summary

Although it is considered to be relatively uncommon complications, GI involvement could pose a significant impact on the BD patient's quality of life due to repeated hospitalizations and even surgeries. Because well-designed therapeutic trials are quite limited, current medical management is empirical and unsatisfactory from both efficacy and safety standpoints. The advent of anti-TNF-α agents could remarkably change our current management and therapeutic goals from relieving symptoms to improved prognosis by achieving mucosal healing.

References

1. Davatchi F, et al. Behcet's disease: from East to West. Clin Rheumatol. 2010;29(8):823–33.
2. Krause I, et al. Childhood Behçet's disease: clinical features and comparison with adult-onset disease. Rheumatology (Oxford). 1999;38(5):457–62.
3. Hung CH, et al. Young children with Behçet disease have more intestinal involvement. J Pediatr Gastroenterol Nutr. 2013;57(2):225–9.
4. Mori S, et al. Esophageal involvement in Behcet's disease. Am J Gastroenterol. 1983;78(9):548–53.
5. Houman MH, et al. Esophageal involvement in Behcet's disease. Yonsei Med J. 2002;43(4):457–60.
6. Ning-Sheng L, Ruay-Sheng L, Kuo-Chih T. High frequency of unusual gastric/duodenal ulcers in patients with Behçet's disease in Taiwan: a possible correlation of MHC molecules with the development of gastric/duodenal ulcers. Clin Rheumatol. 2005;24(5):516–20.
7. Ozenç A, Bayraktar Y, Baykal A. Pyloric stenosis with esophageal involvement in Behçet's syndrome. Am J Gastroenterol. 1990;85(6):727–8.
8. Satake K, et al. Pyloric stenosis: an unusual complication of Behçet's disease. Am J Gastroenterol. 1986;81(9):816–8.
9. Arendt T, et al. A case of Behçet's syndrome presenting with Dieulafoy's ulcer. Z Gastroenterol. 1997;35(10):935–8.
10. Cakmak SK, et al. Upper gastrointestinal abnormalities and Helicobacter pylori in Behçet's disease. Int J Dermatol. 2009;48(11):1174–6.
11. Rhee SH, Kim YB, Lee ES. Comparison of Behcet's disease and recurrent aphthous ulcer according to characteristics of gastrointestinal symptoms. J Korean Med Sci. 2005;20(6):971–6.
12. Ersoy O, et al. H pylori infection in patients with Behcet's disease. World J Gastroenterol. 2007;13(21):2983–5.
13. Kim JS, et al. Prediction of the clinical course of Behçet's colitis according to macroscopic classification by colonoscopy. Endoscopy. 2000;32(8):635–40.
14. Lee SK, et al. Differential diagnosis of intestinal Behçet's disease and Crohn's disease by colonoscopic findings. Endoscopy. 2009;41(1):9–16.
15. Tunç R, et al. A reassessment of the International Study Group criteria for the diagnosis (classification) of Behçet's syndrome. Clin Exp Rheumatol. 2001;19(5 Suppl 24):S45–7.
16. Köklü S, et al. Ileocolonic involvement in Behçet's disease: endoscopic and histological evaluation. Digestion. 2010;81(4):214–7.
17. You JK, et al. Intestinal Behçet's disease: breath-hold MR imaging. Abdom Imaging. 2001;26(3):309–14.
18. Hamdulay SS, et al. Wireless capsule endoscopy in the investigation of intestinal Behçet's syndrome. Rheumatology (Oxford). 2008;47(8):1231–4.
19. Neves FS, et al. Behçet's disease: clinical value of the video capsule endoscopy for small intestine examination. Rheumatol Int. 2009;29(5):601–3.
20. Cheon JH, Korean IBD Study Group, et al. Development, validation, and responsiveness of a novel disease activity index for intestinal Behçet's disease. Inflamm Bowel Dis. 2011;17(2):605–13.
21. Lee HJ, et al. Correlations between endoscopic and clinical disease activity indices in intestinal Behcet's disease. World J Gastroenterol. 2012;18(40):5771–8.
22. Kobayashi M, et al. Neutrophil and endothelial cell activation in the vasa vasorum in vasculo-Behçet disease. Histopathology. 2000;36(4):362–71.
23. Bayraktar Y, et al. Arterial thrombosis leading to intestinal infarction in a patient with Behçet's disease associated with protein C deficiency. Am J Gastroenterol. 1998;93(12):2556–8.
24. Chubachi A, et al. Case report: intestinal infarction after an aneurysmal occlusion of superior mesenteric artery in a patient with Behçet's disease. Am J Med Sci. 1993;306(6):376–8.

25. Hatemi G, EULAR Expert Committee, et al. EULAR recommendations for the management of Behçet disease. Ann Rheum Dis. 2008;67(12):1656–62.
26. Sonta T, et al. The beneficial effect of mesalazine on esophageal ulcers in intestinal Behcet's disease. J Clin Gastroenterol. 2000;30(2):195–9.
27. Yi SW, et al. The prevalence and clinical characteristics of esophageal involvement in patients with Behçet's disease: a single center experience in Korea. J Korean Med Sci. 2009;24(1):52–6.
28. Avci O, et al. Helicobacter pylori and Behçet's disease. Dermatology. 1999;199(2):140–3.
29. Hisamatsu T, et al. The 2nd edition of consensus statements for the diagnosis and management of intestinal Behçet's disease: indication of anti-TNFα monoclonal antibodies. J Gastroenterol. 2014;49(1):156–62.
30. Jung YS, et al. Long-term clinical outcomes and factors predictive of relapse after 5-aminosalicylate or sulfasalazine therapy in patients with intestinal Behcet disease. J Clin Gastroenterol. 2012;46(5):e38–45.
31. Jung YS, et al. Clinical outcomes and prognostic factors for thiopurine maintenance therapy in patients with intestinal Behcet's disease. Inflamm Bowel Dis. 2012;18(4):750–7.
32. Choi IJ, et al. Long-term clinical course and prognostic factors in intestinal Behçet's disease. Dis Colon Rectum. 2000;43(5):692–700.
33. Iwata S, et al. Efficacy of combination therapy of anti-TNF-α antibody infliximab and methotrexate in refractory entero-Behçet's disease. Mod Rheumatol. 2011;21(2):184–91.
34. Hassard PV, et al. Anti-tumor necrosis factor monoclonal antibody therapy for gastrointestinal Behçet's disease: a case report. Gastroenterology. 2001;120(4):995–9.
35. Travis SP, et al. Treatment of intestinal Behçet's syndrome with chimeric tumour necrosis factor alpha antibody. Gut. 2001;49(5):725–8.
36. Kram MT, et al. Behçet's ileocolitis: successful treatment with tumor necrosis factor-alpha antibody (infliximab) therapy: report of a case. Dis Colon Rectum. 2003;46(1):118–21.
37. Byeon JS, et al. Antitumor necrosis factor-alpha therapy for early postoperative recurrence of gastrointestinal Behçet's disease: report of a case. Dis Colon Rectum. 2007;50(5):672–6.
38. Ju JH, et al. Successful treatment of life-threatening intestinal ulcer in Behçet's disease with infliximab: rapid healing of Behçet's ulcer with infliximab. Clin Rheumatol. 2007;26(8):1383–5.
39. Naganuma M, et al. Efficacy of infliximab for induction and maintenance of remission in intestinal Behçet's disease. Inflamm Bowel Dis. 2008;14(9):1259–64.
40. Lee JH, et al. Efficacy of infliximab in intestinal Behçet's disease: a Korean multicenter retrospective study. Inflamm Bowel Dis. 2013;19(9):1833–8.
41. Ariyachaipanich A, Berkelhammer C, Nicola H. Intestinal Behçet's disease: maintenance of remission with adalimumab monotherapy. Inflamm Bowel Dis. 2009;15(12):1769–71.
42. Yasui K, et al. Thalidomide for treatment of intestinal involvement of juvenile-onset Behçet disease. Inflamm Bowel Dis. 2008;14(3):396–400.
43. Iida M, et al. Postoperative recurrence in patients with intestinal Behçet's disease. Dis Colon Rectum. 1994;37(1):16–21.
44. Matsukawa M, et al. Endoscopic therapy with absolute ethanol for postoperative recurrent ulcers in intestinal Behçet's disease, and simple ulcers. J Gastroenterol. 2001;36(4):255–8.
45. Jung YS, et al. Clinical course of intestinal Behcet's disease during the first five years. Dig Dis Sci. 2013;58(2):496–503.
46. Jung YS, et al. Influence of age at diagnosis and sex on clinical course and long-term prognosis of intestinal Behcet's disease. Inflamm Bowel Dis. 2012;18(6):1064–71.
47. Jung YS, et al. Prognostic factors and long-term clinical outcomes for surgical patients with intestinal Behcet's disease. Inflamm Bowel Dis. 2011;17(7):1594–602.

Chapter 8
Mucocutaneous Manifestations

Fumio Kaneko, Ari Togashi, Erika Nomura, and Koichiro Nakamura

Abstract Behçet's disease (BD) is a systemic disorder characterized by recurrent involvement of mucocutaneous, ocular, intestinal, vascular, and/or nervous system organs. We here reviewed the mucocutaneous manifestations including recurrent aphthous stomatitis (RAS) and the several important advances in our understanding of BD pathogenesis based on the genetically intrinsic and extrinsic triggering factors. Most of BD patients tend to have hypersensitivity against oral streptococci which might be acquired through the innate immune mechanism in RAS lesions as one of the extrinsic triggering factors. It was also discussed that the skin prick with self-saliva including oral streptococci was more sensitive than "pathergy test" conventionally used for BD diagnosis. HLA-B51-restricted $CD8^{+}$ T cell response is suspected to be correlated with the target tissues expressing major histocompatibility complex class I chain-related gene A (MICA) by stress in active BD patients as the intrinsic factors. *Bes-1* gene and 65kD of heat shock protein (HSP-65) derived from oral *Streptococcus sanguinis* (*S. sanguinis)* are supposed to play an important role as the extrinsic factor in BD pathogenesis. The peptides of *Bes-1* gene are highly homologous with the retinal protein *Brn3b*, and moreover they are also homology with HSP-65 in association with the counterpart human HSP-60 which reactively appeared in serum of the patients. The HSP-65/60 also has the high homologies with the respective T cell epitope of BD patients. Then, the pathogenesis of BD was conclusively discussed on the relationship between RAS and the systemic symptoms by the vascular reaction due to immune responses against oral *S. sanguinis* agents.

Keywords Behçet's disease • Mucocutaneous manifestation • Heat shock protein • *Streptococcus sanguinis* • Vascular reaction

---

F. Kaneko, M.D. (✉) • A. Togashi, Ph.D. • E. Nomura, M.D.
Institute of Dermato-Immunology and Allergy, Southern TOHOKU Research Institute for Neuroscience, Koriyama, Fukushima, Japan
e-mail: f.kaneko@mt.strins.or.jp; ari_ha_belluga_suki@yahoo.c.jp; erika_berry@yahoo.c.jp

K. Nakamura, M.D., Ph.D.
Department of Dermatology, Saitama Medical University, Saitama, Japan
e-mail: nakamu@saitama-med.ac.jp

Y. Ishigatsubo (ed.), *Behçet's Disease*,
DOI 10.1007/978-4-431-54487-6_8

8.1 Introduction

Behçet's disease (BD) [1] is a chronic systemic inflammatory disorder characterized by the recurrent involvement of mucocutaneous [*recurrent aphthous stomatitis (RAS)*, genital ulceration, erythema nodosum (EN)-like eruption, acne-like eruption, etc.], ocular, vascular, digestive, and/or nervous system organs. Although the actual etiology of BD is still unclear, the pathogenesis has been generally clearer by the etiological research based on the genetically intrinsic factors and immunological reactions by the extrinsic triggering factors [2–13]. As one of the triggering factors, the oral unhygienic condition may be suspected, because periodontitis, decayed teeth, chronic tonsillitis, etc., are frequently noted in the oral cavity of BD patients [9, 10]. The proportion of *Streptococcus sanguinis (S. sanguinis)*, which was previously recognized as *species* of the *genus Streptococcus* named "*S. sanguis*," was significantly high in the oral bacterial flora of BD patients in comparison with those of healthy controls. *S. sanguinis* from BD patients was identified as uncommon serotype KTH-1 (so-called BD113-20) by the bacterial and enzymatic properties [11–13]. Most of BD patients tend to acquire hypersensitivity against *streptococci* in their oral flora, as previously demonstrated that the cutaneous reactions by the intracutaneous injection and/or prickle tests with bacteria antigens of *streptococci* and *enterococci,* except for *staphylococci,* were much stronger than the reaction by "pathergy test" [8, 9, 14, 15]. Non-BD patients with RAS were also reported to react with streptococcal antigen [16]. In vitro system, inflammatory cytokines, interleukin (IL)-6, and interferon (IFN)-γ were produced from peripheral blood mononuclear cells (PBMCs) of BD patients by stimulation with streptococcal antigen [17]. The titers of serum-antibody against *streptococci* were also elevated in BD patients [18]. The 65 kDa of heat shock protein (HSP-65) derived from oral *S. sanguinis* can be detected along with counterpart human HSP-60 which reactively appears in the sera and lesions of BD patients. The peptides of HSP-65 derived from *streptococci* show considerable homology with those of the human HSP-60 [19–21].

Then, we have attempted to review on the mucocutaneous manifestations and a new diagnostic way in the connection with the immunopathology based on the genetically intrinsic and extrinsic triggering factors in BD patients.

8.2 Mucocutaneous Involvements (Fig. 8.1a–f)

8.2.1 RAS

RAS showing oral aphthous ulceration generally starts as an initial symptom in BD patients since childhood and/or youth (Fig. 8.1a, b) and other mucocutaneous symptoms follow [22–24]. The oral aphthous ulceration, which is like a punch-out shape, occurs with pain on the tongue, buccal mucosa, gingival, and lip in BD

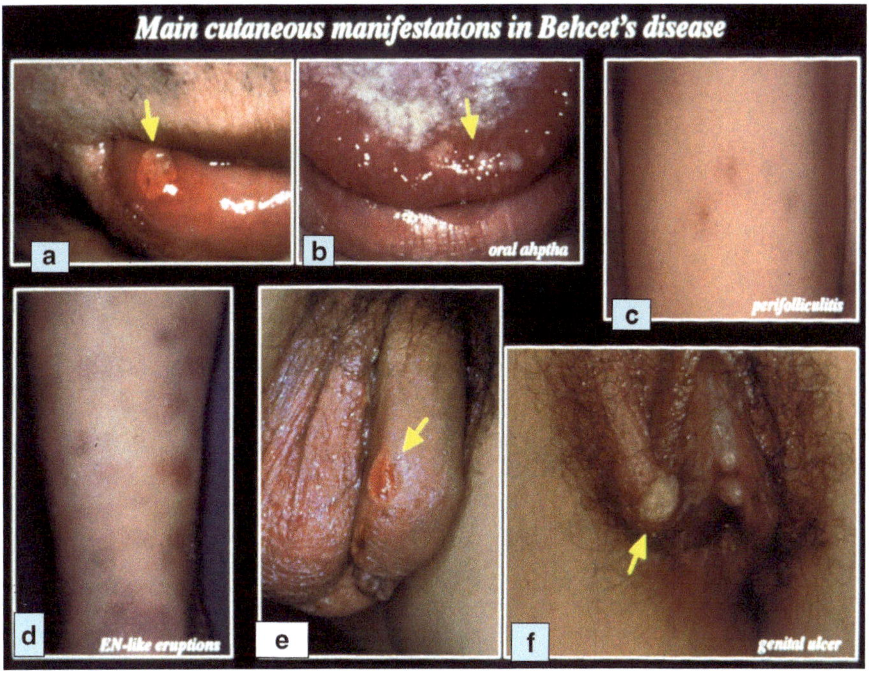

Fig. 8.1 Clinical features of mucocutaneous symptoms in BD patients. (**a**) Major type of aphthous ulceration (recurrent aphthous stomatitis (RAS) lesion) on the lower lip (*arrow*). (**b**) Herpetiform stomatitis of the tongue (*arrow*). (**c**) Acne-like eruption (perifolliculitis). (**d**) Erythema nodosum (EN)-like eruption. (**e**) Penile ulceration (*arrow*). (**f**) Female genital ulceration (*arrow*)

patients, and it continues around a week. The clinical classification of the oral ulcers is divided as minor, major, herpetiform, and the combined types by lesional size and shapes. However, non-BD-RAS is a very common disorder due to trauma, some viral and/or bacterial infections, and other autoimmune diseases, because it is known that 20 % of the general population is affected in the world [25]. All RAS patients are not BD, but nearly 100 % of BD patients are associated with RAS [22–24]. The biopsy specimen of aphthous ulcer lesion from a BD patient revealed a reaction like the antibody-dependent cell-mediated cytotoxicity showing that the epithelial cells surrounded by neutrophils and lymphoid cells (Fig. 8.2a, b) and that they look like leaves falling down from the mucous epithelial layer, which can be seen by the smear cells (Fig. 8.2c). These epithelial cells were stained with antihuman IgA, IgM, complement, streptococcal antibodies, and HLA-DR monoclonal antibody, and they are surrounded by T cells in the immunohistology [14, 26]. However, it is difficult to differentiate BD from non-BD-RAS by the clinically morphological findings, because this histology is not a specific feature of BD-RAS.

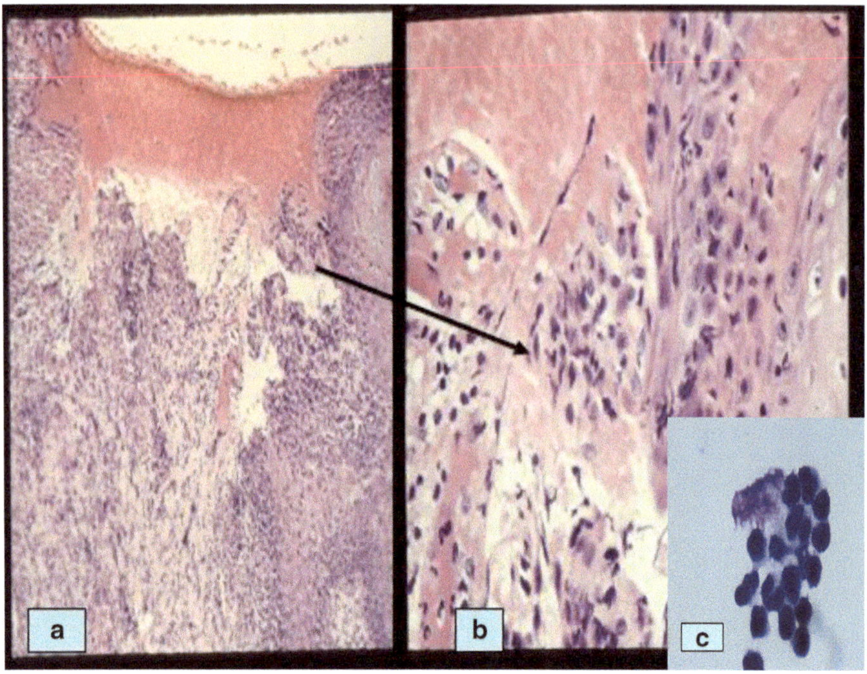

Fig. 8.2 Histology of aphthous ulceration of a BD patient. (**a**) Aphthous ulceration of the lip, showing lack of the epithelial layer and in the ulcer bottom a numerous inflammatory cell infiltration (HE, ×100). (**b**) Magnified feature of the ulcer edge of the epithelial layer. The epithelial cells are surrounded by inflammatory infiltrates (HE, ×400). (**c**). Smear cell form the aphthous ulcer showing "Rosetta formation" (Giemsa stain, ×400)

8.2.2 Genital Ulcer

The clinical features of genital ulceration are generally shaped as similar to oral aphthous ulceration (Fig. 8.1e, f). Sometimes the young female patients are suddenly attacked by genital ulceration as the initial BD symptom clinically like Lipschutz ulceration [27]. Some female BD patients develop to show genital large ulcerations [28]. About more than 50 % of BD patients are found to be associated with genital ulceration (female: 55.5 %, male: 58.7 %), that is, ulcers occur on the vulva (66.1 %), vaginal mucosa (35.7 %), anus (9.6 %), cervix (4.1), and groin area (0.8 %) in female patients and on the penis (46.5 %), scrotum (38.5 %), anus (9.2 %), and groin area (5.0 %) in male patients [22, 24].

8.2.3 EN-Like Eruption

More than 50 % of BD patients are reported to be associated with EN-like eruption on the lower legs [22–24], which looks relatively smaller than "erythematous indulation" of non-BD patients (Figs. 8.1d, 8.4a). The histology is generally vascular reaction

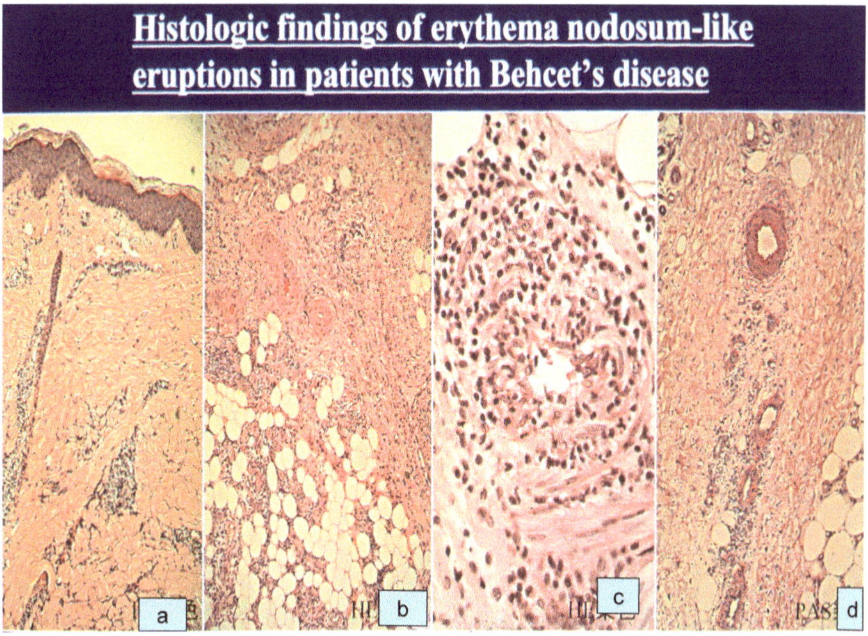

Fig. 8.3 Histology of EN-like eruption. (**a**) Perivascular infiltration by lymphoid cells in the upper and deep dermis (HE, ×100). (**b**) So-called septal panniculitis in the subcutaneous tissue (HE, ×100). (**c**) Perivascular infiltration, so-called lymphocytic vasculitis (HE, ×400). (**d**) Necrotizing vasculitis can be also seen in the part of perivascular infiltration (PAS reaction, ×200)

infiltrated by mainly lymphoid cells, so-called lymphocytic vasculitis, and septal panniculitis in the subcutaneous fatty tissue (Fig. 8.3a–d). In acute phase, however, vasculitis surrounded by neutrophils is able to be recognized. Immunofluorescence revealed deposits of IgA, IgM, complement in the vascular walls and streptococcal-related materials can be also detected in the vascular walls by antistreptococcal antibody (Fig. 8.4a–c) [9, 14, 26]. The findings suggest that streptococcal antigens might be playing an important role as the triggering extrinsic factor, as mentioned previously [8, 9, 14, 26]. Recently, Korian research group have demonstrated that GroEL of *S. sanguinis* and human heterogenous nuclear ribonucleoprotein (hnRNP)A2/B1 were expressed on the vascular walls in EN-like eruption of BD patients [29, 30].

8.2.4 Other Mucocutaneous Disorders

Acne-like eruption due to perifolliculitis repeatedly appears on the upper body of BD patients and subcutaneous thrombophlebitis, so-called thrombophlebitis migrans, is suddenly noticed on the lower extremities. Rarely the follicular lesions develop to large ulcerations like "pyoderma gangrenosum" on the extremities. Some male BD patients have edema of the scrotum with sudden pain due to epididymitis.

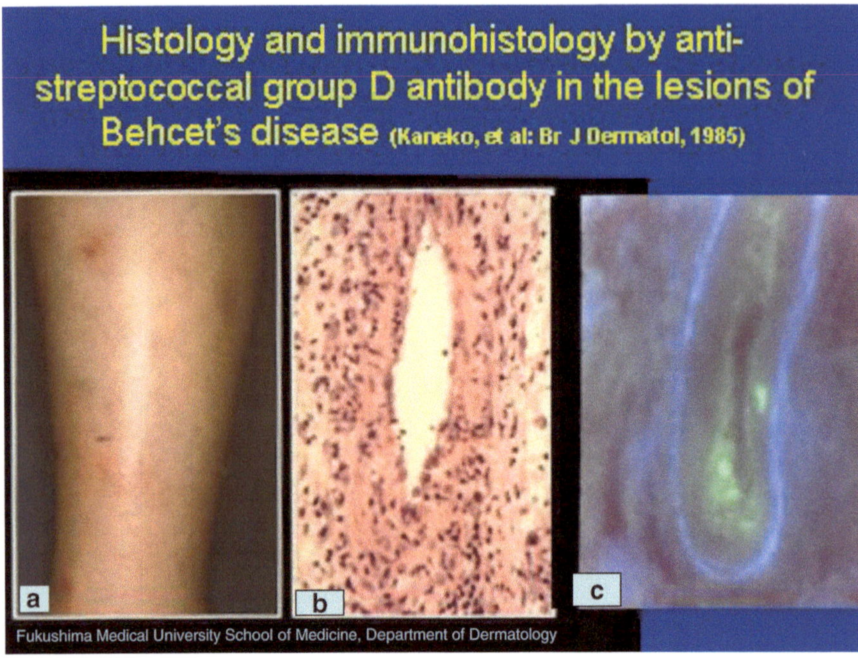

Fig. 8.4 Histology and immunohistology of "vasculitis" of EN-like eruption by antistreptococcal antibody [9, 14]. (**a**) EN-like eruption of a BD patient. (**b**) Vasculitis infiltrated by lymphoid cells and a few neutrophils in EN-like eruption (HE, ×400). (**c**) Deposits of streptococcal antigen and its bearing cells adhering to the vascular wall (direct immunofluorescence by antistreptococcal antibody, ×400)

8.3 Pathergy Test and Oral Streptococci

It is not difficult to make a diagnosis for BD except for the atypical cases without the main mucocutaneous symptoms including RAS. Pathergy test, which is a nonspecific cutaneous hypersensitive reaction showing around 2 mm pustule 24–48 h after 20G syringe needle stick, has been thought to be helpful to diagnose BD for long time, because the phenomenon has been believed as a unique feature of BD and it is one of diagnostic criteria by International Study Group of Behçet's Disease [31]. Histology and immunohistology of the "pathergy reaction" are similar to those of EN-like eruption of BD patients [32–34]. However, recently the positivity became chronologically lower to less than 40 % of BD patients seen in 2007s, though more than 70 % of the patients showed positive in 1970s. Besides, its diagnostic value is different from the prevalence in the countries [35–37]. It is of interest that the surgical cleaning of the forearm before needle prick reduced its reactivity [38], suggesting that the "pathergy reaction" might be a cutaneous response to some bacteria living on the surface of the skin. Then, instead of "pathergy test," we tried to prick with self-saliva, which oral bacteria including streptococci are ordinary contained (Fig. 8.5), to the forearm of BD patients for diagnosis using Lancetter with tiny stick

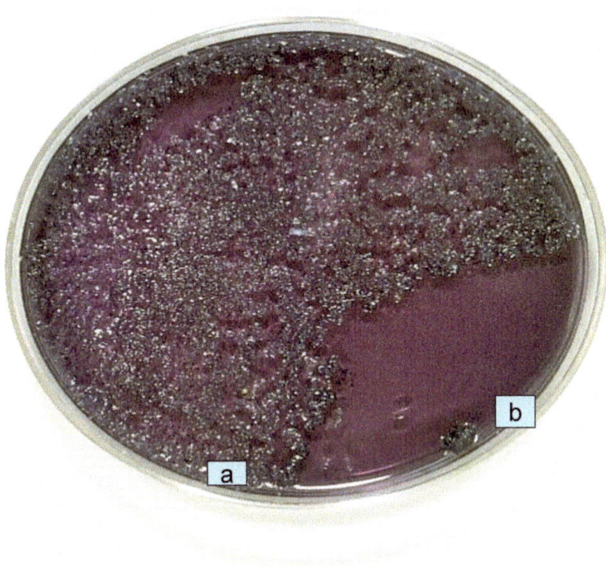

Fig. 8.5 Incubation of saliva from a BD patient in MS (mitis and salivarius) agar which is streptococcus selectively grown. (**a**) Oral streptococci grew from saliva in 5 days. (**b**) Incubation area of the sterilized saliva by a syringe micromembrane filter

Fig. 8.6 Prick test with self-saliva using Lancetter. The skin reactions were observed as erythema of more than 10 mm in diameter with a spot pustule 48 h after prick with pure self-saliva in a 33-year-old female BD patient. *S* self-saliva, *SS* sterilized saliva using syringe filter with 0.2 μm pores, *CS* control saline

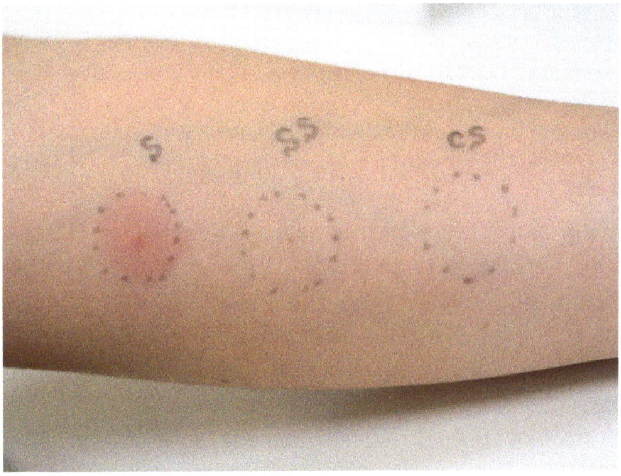

(OY ALGO AB Espoo/Esbo, Sweden), because the patients have hypersensitivity to oral streptococci. The results revealed more than 90 % of 9 BD patients showed erythematous reaction with spot pustule by the stick with self-saliva (Fig. 8.6), and the histology of the positive site was basically similar to that of EN lesions. Non-BD-RAS patients showed weaker reaction than those of BD patients, suggesting to be differentiated from each other. No reaction and/or tiny spot was seen by the prick

Table 8.1 Results of the self-salivary prick tests in BD and non-BD-RAS patients and controls [39]

Age, sex		S-prick test			
Patients (initials)		(after 48 h)	Small pustule	SS-prick	CS-prick
Neuro BD	55 M YY	11×15 mm	+	nd	–
Incomplete	33 F AT[a]	22×22	–	–	–
	26 F MN[a]	10×10	+	+ dot	–
	27 M TG	11×12	+	+ dot	–
	47 M YT	10×13	+	+ dot	–
	36 F AN[a]	5×10	–	nd	–
	46 M KH	10×10	–	–	–
	17 F YT	5×5	–	–	–
Complete	23 M OO[a]	10×10	+	–	–
Recurrent aphthous stomatitis (non-BD-RAS)					
	24 F YN	8×10 mm	–	–	–
	28 F YS	8×4	–	–	–
	32 F YN	–	–	nd	–
	29 M ON	–	–	nd	–
	28 F MS	3×5	–	–	–
Disease controls					
Non-BD EN 39 F KY		–	–	nd	–
61 F MF		–	–		–
Viral aphthosis [3]		–	–	nd	–
Healthy controls [6]		–	–	–	–

Togashi et al. [39]
The clinical type of BD is followed by the Japanese BD classification
BD Behçet's disease, *EN* erythema nodosum, *F* female, *M* male, *nd* not done
[a]Same cases in Table 8.2
S-prick prick with self-saliva, SS-prick prick with sterilized self-saliva, CS-prick prick with saline, dot small spot, + positive, – negative

with microfilter-sterilized saliva and saline in BD patients and controls; patients with viral aphtha and non-BD EN and healthy persons did not show the cutaneous reaction (Table 8.1) [39]. The results also suggest that oral *streptococci* are playing an important role in the pathogenesis of the RAS of BD patients and that the salivary prick is able to make a differentiation of BD from non-BD disorders. The severity of the cutaneous reactions by salivary prick did not seem to be correlated with the possession of HLA-B51 in BD patients, as described later (Table 8.2) [40].

8.4 HLA Genotyping of BD and Streptococcal Infection

HLA-B51 is supposed to be a highly associated genetic marker of BD patients from many different ethnic groups including European, Mediterranean, and Asian people and BD has several unique epidemiologic features which seem to go from Southern

Table 8.2 Self-salivary prick test in BD patients with and without HLA-B51 [40]

Type of BD	Patients (initials)	Prick test (mm)			HLA-B51
(Japanese classification)		S	SS	CS	
Complete type	23 M OO[a]	10	–	–	+ (B51)
Intestinal type	37 F NI	20	2	–	+ (B51, 52)
Incomplete type	40 M HG	10	7	–	+ (B51, 01, 01)
	31 F MA	30	7	–	+ (B51, 40)
	42 F MK	7	4	–	+ (B51, 46, DR4, 8)
Incomplete type	34 F MY	26	5	–	–(B35, 48)
	36 F AN[a]	10	–	–	–(B44, 03, 01)
	33 F YK	10	–	–	–
	37 F AT[a]	22	–	–	–(B40, 48)
	30 F MN[a]	10	–	–	–
	35 M YI	10	nd	–	–(B15, 35)
	37 F HT	4	–	–	–(B40, 44)
	36 M MK	4	3	–	–(B35, 44)
	35 M KF	7	2	–	–(B46, 54)
	35 F YO	14	–	–	–(B07, 02, 01)

F female, *M* male, *S* self-saliva, *SS* filtered sterilized saliva, *CS* control saline, *nd* not done
+ positive, – negative
[a]Same cases in Table 8.1

Europe to Japan along "the old Silk Road"[2, 4, 5, 41, 42]. The appearance of BD lesions is not directly correlated with HLA-B51 in the immunological background of the patients, but it was found that HLA-B51-restricted cytotoxic T lymphocytes (CTLs) played some roles in correlation with the stressed target tissues expressing major histocompatibility complex class I chain-related gene A (MICA) in BD pathogenesis. When the transmembrane MICA nearly located at the HLA-B51 gene is preferentially expressed on epithelial and endothelial cells by stress, they seem to be the candidates for the HLA-B51-restricted CTLs response, and MICA expressed on the stressed epithelium and endothelium is considered to be the ligand for activating natural killer (NK) cells with NKG2D molecule and CD8$^+$T cells as CTLs [43, 44]. Regarding NK cell activation, inhibitory CD34/NKG2A and activating CD94/NKG2C molecules are alternatively expressed on NK, CD4 $^+$CD8 $^+$T cells, as indicating an imbalance in cytotoxic activity in BD patients [45]. However, the function of NK cells is supposed to be downregulated in the active stage and to be upregulated in the remission of BD patients [46]. The expressive CD4$^+$T cells activated by inflammatory cytokines including interferon (IFN)-γ, IL-12, IL-23, etc., might be altered to Th17 cells, which release IL-17 in the BD lesions, as seen in autoimmune disorders [47, 48].

It is also considered that HSP-65/60 derived from microorganism including *S. sanguinis* and the damaged human tissues, which is actually detectable in the oral mucosal and skin lesions of BD patients, also becomes a stress-inducible factor in connection with MICA*009 expression [19, 20]. Generally, it has been reported that antigen-presenting cells (APCs) expressing IL-12 are thought to be activated in BD patients with HLA-B51 in active stage [41]. However, we have obtained interesting results that PBMCs from BD patients without HLA-B51 gene can be significantly stimulated by *S. sanguinis* antigen in the expression of IL-12p40 mRNA and increasing of protein level in connection with IL-12p70 (70 kDa composed of p35 and p40 subunits) rather than those of the patients with HLA-B51 [49]. It has been suggested that antibacterial host response in T cell type immunity mediated by IL-12 is much stronger in HLA-B51-negative BD patients in vitro experiment. The cutaneous reactions by prick test with self-saliva also showed no difference between BD patients with and without HLA-B51 in vivo responses (Table 8.2), as seen in those of pathergy test, reported previously [36, 40].

8.5 Hypersensitivity Against *S. sanguinis*

Generally, the oral health is impaired in BD patients who seem to be associated with the disease severity [8–10, 12, 13]. It is not clear that the predisposition of BD patients may be correlated with streptococcal infection due to defect of the bactericidal effects, but the uncommon serotype oral *S. sanguinis* is significantly increased in BD patients compared with healthy and disease controls [11–13]. The antibodies against *S. sanguinis* in sera from BD patients showed cross-reactivity with some synthetic peptides of HSP-65 derived from *S. sanguinis* [50, 51]. The patients show strong delayed-type cutaneous hypersensitivity reactions against streptococcal antigens in skin tests, and sometimes the BD symptoms were provoked by skin injection of the antigens [8, 9, 14, 15]. Because aphthous ulceration can be also induced by a prick with streptococcal antigen on the oral mucous membrane of a BD patient [9, 15], RAS is considered to be due to the hypersensitive reaction against *oral streptococci* when they are traumatically penetrated into the oral membrane. Isogai et al. [51] demonstrated that the symptoms mimicking BD appeared in germ-free mice when *S. sanguinis* from BD patients was inoculated into their oral tissue damaged by heat shock and/or mechanical stress. This report suggests that the immunization with *S. sanguinis* through the oral membrane route elicits BD-like symptoms in the animal model as seen in BD patients who carry *S. sanguinis* as the pathogenic microorganism in their oral cavity. We tried to find polymerase chain reaction (PCR) targeting *Bes-1* gene in BD lesions using two distinct primer sets (peptides, 229-243 and 373-385) encoding *S. sanguinis* (serotype KTH-1) which was prepared by Yoshikawa et al. [52]. *Bes-1* DNA was present in various mucocutaneous lesions including oral and genital ulcerations and EN-like lesions, and the PCR in situ hybridization revealed that *Bes-1* DNA was expressed in the cytoplasm of inflammatory infiltrated monocytes adhering the vascular walls in mucocutaneous lesions (Fig. 8.7) [53]. In contrast, we failed to detect DNAs of herpes simplex virus (HSV)-1, HSV-2, cytomegalovirus, human herpes virus (HHV)-6, and HHV-7 in the lesions by PCR [54], although HSV infection has been speculated as etiologically important since the report of H. Behcet [1]. However, the animal models infected by HSV have been also demonstrated to mimic BD-like symptoms [55]. Interestingly, the amino acid sequence of the peptides of *Bes-1* (229-243 and 373-385) shows more

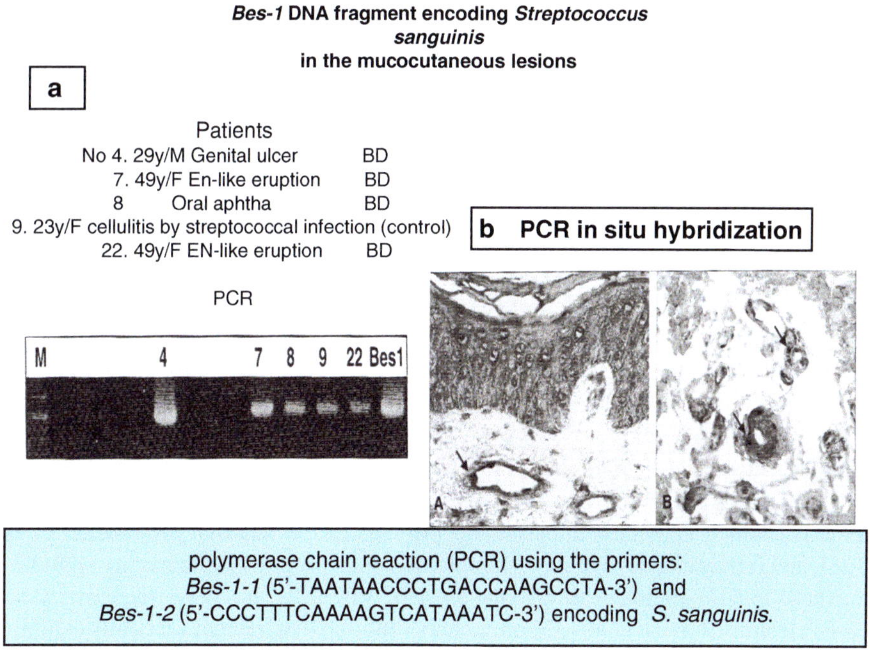

Fig. 8.7 *Bes-1* gene expression in the mucocutaneous lesions of patients with BD [53]. (**a**). Three of 11 BD patients were positive for *Bes-1* DNA in the lesions including aphthous and genital ulcerations and erythema nodosum (EN)-like eruption by amplified polymerase chain reaction (PCR) using the primers: *Bes-1-1* (5′-TAATAACCCTGACCAAGCCTA-3′-) and *Bes-1-2* (5′-CCCTTTCAAAAGTCATAAATC-3′) encoding *S. sanguinis*. (**b**) In these positive lesions, *Bes-1* DNA was also detected in the cytoplasm of monocytes adhering to the vascular walls and infiltrated around the vessels by PCR in situ hybridization

than 60 % similarity to the human intraocular ganglion peptide, *Brn-3b*, which is a subfamily of POU (pit-Oct Unc) domain factors containing *Brn-3a* and *Brn-3c* [56]. The peptide of *Bes-1* (229-243) was also found to be correlated with the peptide of HSP-60 (336-351) [50]. Recently it was found that the peptide of *Bes-1* (337-385) stimulated PBMCs of BD patients in production of IFN-γ and IL-12, though the cellular proliferation was not observed [57]. These results suggest that *Bes-1* derived from oral *S. sanguinis* might be an inducer for the possible retinal and neural involvement in BD patients.

8.6 HSP-65 Derived from Microorganism and Human HSP-60

HSPs, which scavenge denatured intracellular proteins, are supposed to be induced by microorganisms and mammalian tissues under a variety of stressful condition [58], and they may be involved in the pathogenesis of some autoimmune diseases

[59]. In BD patients, the serum levels of IgA antibodies to mycobacterial HSP-65, which cross-reacts with selected strains of *S. sanguinis*, are significantly increased [59, 60]. HSPs taken up by APCs are thought to stimulate T cells directly, the monocytes expressing HSP-60 lead T cells to undergo apoptosis after IFN-γ production [64], and the presence of HSP-60 was also detected in various lesions of BD patients [61–63]. On the other hand, 4 peptides of HSP-65 (111-125, 154-172, 219-233, and 311-326) derived from *S. sanguinis* were recognized as immunodominant agents for T and B cell responses, and they showed 50–80 % homology to the counterpart human HSP-60 [20, 63–65]. The 4 peptides of HSP-65 were shown to significantly stimulate and undergo $CD4^+$ and $CD8^+$ T cell apoptosis in PBMCs from BD patients, and HSP-60 also seemed to stimulate them [61, 62]. On the contrary, the other two peptides of HSP-65 (21-35 and 401-415) corresponding to the peptide of human HSP-60 (425-441) are reported not to stimulate PBMCs from BD patients and healthy individuals [58]. The peptide of HSP-60 (336-351) was also identified to be highly homologous to T cell epitope [58, 60–67]. Whole HSP-60 is, however, suspected to induce vascular endothelial growth factor (VEGF) which activates, impairs, and propagates the vascular endothelial cells [68], and it may also lead to thrombophlebitis and vasculitis by damaging endothelial cells in BD patients. Although the term of "vasculitis" has been frequently used in BD lesions, Jorrizo et al. [33] previously reported that the real vasculitis exhibiting "necrotizing vasculitis" was rarely seen in EN-like eruption of BD patients and, in most cases, the vascular reaction surrounded by monocytes and a few neutrophils that is so-called lymphocytic vasculitis seen histologically, as recently described by other authors [69, 70]. It is observed, however, that the serum levels of soluble(s) adhesion molecules, such as s-selectins and s-intercellular adhesion molecule-1, are elevated [71, 72] and also the expression of VEGF is increased in the presence of HSP in the lesions of BD [73]. The subcutaneous administration of HSP peptides to the mice has been shown to induce uveitis with vascular impairment [74].

On the other hand, it is of interest that the peptide of HSP-60 (336-351) linked to recombinant cholera toxin B subunit (rCTB) reduced the uveitis induced by whole HSP-60, although the peptide without adjuvant is reported to induce uveitis in Lewis strain rats [74, 75]. A therapeutic trial by the peptide conjugated with rCTB was performed as it was orally given to BD patients with recurrent uveitis. The successful results were obtained to show that five of eight patients had no relapse of uveitis and that two of the remaining three patients had improved recurrent oral ulceration, folliculitis, EN-like eruptions, and genital ulcers without any side effects [76]. In those patients with uveitis and extra-articular manifestations, a lack of the peptide-specific $CD4^+$ T cell population, a decrease in expression of Th1-type cells (CCR5, CXCR3), and a reduction of IFN-γ, TNF-α, $CCR7^+$ T cells, and co-stimulatory molecules (CD40 and CD28) were observed in comparison to BD patients with relapse of disease [76]. These findings may suggest immuno-torelation in active BD patients. It is hypothesized that CTLs play a role in BD pathogenesis by targeting a self-antigen selectively expressed in the affected tissues. In BD patients with active disease, the endogenously generated MICA transmembrane-peptide by autoreactive CTLs is present [43], and the excessive inflammatory responses might be induced by the extrinsic factors correlated with *S. sanguinis* and other organisms including *Helicobacter pylori*, *Mycoplasma fermentas,* etc. [77–79]. Neutrophilic hyperfunction and a cross-reactive autoimmune response between microbial and human HSPs are proposed to be correlated with the hyperreactivity against microorganism including *S. sanguinis* in BD patients [8, 9, 14, 15, 17]. These HSPs presented by APCs can directly stimulate $\alpha\beta^{+}$T and $\gamma\delta^{+}$ T cells which play important roles in the oral mucosal immunity as the first defense against microorganisms. It is thought that $V\gamma9\delta2^{+}$ T cells, a major subset of $\gamma\delta^{+}$ T cells in PBMCs, recognize antigens produced by bacteria and that innate and adaptive immune responses were influenced by secreting IFN-γ, towards a Th1 profile [80]. These $\gamma\delta^{+}$ T cells seemed to be elevated in PBMCs and in the mucocutaneous lesions of BD patients [81]. The second major subset, $\gamma\delta1^{+}$ T cell, is enriched in the mucosa, and the antigens are presented by APCs with stress-inducible MICA and MICB. The $\gamma\delta^{+}$T cells which highly express CD29 and CD69 produce IFN-γ and TNF-α from stimulation by HSP-65/60 in the peripheral blood and in the lesions of BD patients with active disease [20, 62]. These activated APCs and $\gamma\delta^{+}$T cells might activate $\alpha\beta^{+}$T cells by their secretion of sIL-2R, IFN-γ, and TNF-α and also high levels of other cytokines, IL-1α, IL-6, IL-8, IL-15, etc., which are detected in sera of BD patients [81–83]. In the active stage of BD patients, IL-12 is also produced as a sign of Th1 type reaction advanced. The gene polymorphism in the promoter region regarding a 4 bp insertion within IL-12p40 was significantly higher in the HLA-B51-negative BD patients than HLA-B51-positive patients and healthy individuals. The expression of IL-12p40 mRNA and protein levels in conjugation with IL-12p70 induction were also significantly increased in PBMCs from BD patients without HLA-B51 by stimulation with *S. sanguinis* antigen [49], and the expression of IL-23, which is composed of a shared p40 subunit of IL-12 and p19 subunit of IL-23, was also increased with IL-12 in EN-like lesions of BD patients [84].

Although antibodies against the HSP peptides derived from bacteria including *S. sanguinis* are found in sera of BD patients [50, 51], HSP-specific antibodies and T cells are considered to play a complicated role in the pathogenesis of human autoimmune diseases [85]. HSPs might trigger both innate and adaptive immune mechanisms in BD. On the other hand, the therapeutic approaches involving HSP immunomodulation may be available as "oral toleration" using the peptide of HSP (336-351) linked to rCTB for BD patients with advanced *uveitis*, as demonstrated by Stanford et al. [76]. In order to understand the suppressive mechanisms of the cytokine production in PBMCs from active BD patients, we tried to find the binding sites of the peptides on monocytes by cDNA chips (Gene Chip; Human Genome) using NOMO-1 cells (human macrophage cell line) activated by *S. sanguinis* antigen, and they were incubated with the peptides. It was found that although the expression of IL-8, IL-16, IL-13R, and IL-17R was decreased after incubation with LO1 and UK, respectively, LO2 did not decrease IL-8 production. CD58 (lymphocyte function-associated antigen-3) molecule and/or FK506 binding protein were highly expressed on the cell membrane after application of LO1 and UK [86, 87].

8.7 Toll-Like Receptor (TLR) Expression in the Innate Immunity

Regarding the recognition system for the microorganism antigens in humans, ten numbers of TLR family are supposed to act as innate immune receptors by binding of particular structures present on bacteria, viruses, fungi, etc. [88]. Although generally TLRs are weakly detectable in various human tissues with varying levels, the TLR expression of the organs involved in immune response and exposed to environment is found to be significantly stronger [89]. TLR-3 [ds RNA] and TLR-6 [mycoplasma, staphylococci, etc.] are also reported to be enhanced in expression on neutrophils and monocytes of BD patients, when stimulated by HSP-60 and *S. sanguinis* antigen [90]. In RAS lesion, expression of TLR-9 [unmethylated CpG DNA, bacteria, and virus] has been also found [91]. These findings suggest that innate immune system contributes the acquisition of hypersensitivity against oral streptococci in the pathogenesis of BD as the extrinsic factor.

8.8 Complement System in the Innate Immunity

Compliment system is thought to be activated in relation with chemokines and neutrophilic activation regarding innate immunity [92, 93]. Deposits of complement C3 with immunoglobulins are frequently detectable by immunofluorescent techniques in BD lesions [14, 26, 70]. With respect to the complement system of BD patients, the titer of serum complement is generally high in the inactive stage but decreases in the active stage, although the levels of mannose-binding lectin (MBL) pathway are decreased [94]. The MBL pathway is considered to play an important role in the innate immunity. A C-type serum lectin secreted by the liver binds to mannose and N-acetyl-glucosamine oligosaccharides on the surfaces of yeast, bacteria, and viruses, and the reaction serves as the initiator of the third pathway of the complement system in independent from antibodies [95]. Ficolin (FCN) is a soluble protein that binds to carbohydrate on the microbial cells and 3 different types of FCN are detected. FCN 1 and 2 genes are located in the chromosome 9q34 and FCN3 gene is assigned to chromosome 1. FCN 2 binds to lipoteichoic acid on the cell wall constituent in all Gram-positive bacteria and activate immune cells to produce proinflammatory cytokines [92, 96]. We have found that novel FCN 2 gene single nucleotide polymorphisms (SNPs) are identified in the promoter regions as well as in the exon regions. The MBL genetic polymorphisms might be involved in immune responses to streptococcus infections in BD patients, because the relationship between MBL gene mutations and microbiological factors was suspected in the lesional immune reaction of BD patients [97]. Although no significant difference was present in the genotype allele frequencies of MBL gene SNPs between BD patients and healthy controls, the allele frequencies of FCN2 gene SNPs were significantly recognized in the promoter regions (-557 and -64 sites) among HLA-B51-positive BD patients [98]. The findings suggest the possibility that FCN gene of the MBL pathway in complement system contributes to the innate immunity in BD patients.

8.9 RAS and Systemic Symptoms

BD symptoms are characterized by vascular involvements histologically showing swollen endothelial cells of the micro-arteries infiltrated by inflammatory monocytes and a few neutrophils, as seen in so-called vascular reaction of EN-like eruption and other lesions [14, 33, 69, 70]. The strong hypersensitivity reaction against *S. sanguinis* agents, which might be gained by APCs through the innate immune mechanism, can be suspected as the extrinsic triggering factor in the pathogenesis of BD [8, 9, 14, 15, 17]. In the treatment by antibiotics for the involvement of oral *S. sanguinis*, especially minocycline, which reduces not only the growth of streptococci but also suppresses IL-1β and IL-6 production from T cells inflamed, was clinically effective for RAS, acne-like eruption, and EN-like lesion in BD patients [9]. Other study also showed that combination therapy, colchicine, and benzathine penicillin was effective to suppress BD symptoms compared to colchicine monotherapy [99, 100]. Mumcu et al. [100] and others [5–7] have already reviewed on the role of infectious agents in BD pathogenesis, but also we dare to propose the hypothesis that after *Bes-1* gene taken in the cytoplasm of APCs through the TLRs in RAS lesion, the APCs, which are expressing the streptococcal antigen, produce HSP-65. If these APCs curried adhere to the impaired and/or MICA-expressed endothelium of the vessels in correlation with HSP-65/60, VEGF, adhesion molecules, etc., BD lesions may be induced by the "vascular reaction" and/or "lymphocytic vasculitis" as the immunological reaction due to the APCs expressing *S. sanguinis* antigen. Then, we would like to express the hypothesis as the correlation between RAS and systemic symptoms in BD patients (Fig. 8.8) [40, 101, 102].

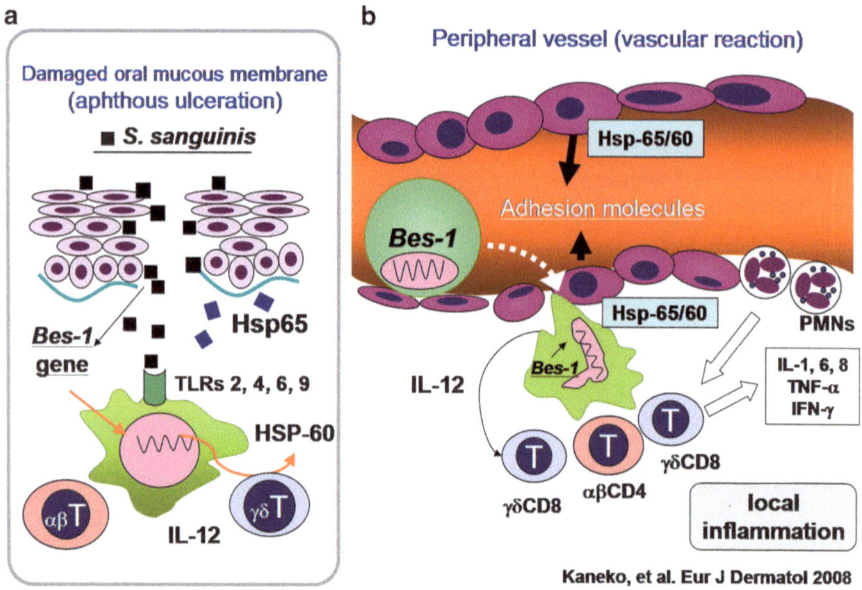

Fig. 8.8 Hypothesis of the correlation between recurrent aphthous stomatitis (RAS) and the peripheral lesions in BD patients. (**a**) The immunization of antigen-presenting cells (APCs) (macrophages and/or dendritic cells) by *S. sanguinis* agents through TLRs in the oral cavity. (**b**) If the APCs are transferred in the blood flow, the immunological reaction might be induced at the impaired and/or MICA and adhesion molecules expressed endothelial cells of vascular wall, as BD lesion

8.10 Conclusion

BD pathogenesis was discussed in the aspects of the genetic intrinsic factors and extrinsic triggering factors. HLA-B51-restricted CTL was found to target the MICA-expressed organs by stress in correlation with HSP-65/60 derived from the oral bacteria including *S. sanguinis*. The immune responses based on Th1-type reaction with chemotaxis by the bacterial agents are considered to correlate with various BD symptoms which were caused by "vascular reaction" and/or "lymphocytic vasculitis" histologically.

Acknowledgments We deeply appreciate that the studies were supported by the grants from the study group of Behçet's disease organized by Japanese Ministry of Health, Labour and Welfare.

References

1. Behcet H. Uber rezidivierende, aphthous durch ein Virus verursachte Geschwuere am Mund, am Auge und an den Genitalien. Dermatol Wochenschr. 1937;105:1152–7.

2. Altenburg A, Papoutsis N, Orawa H, Martus P, Krause L, Zouboulis CC. Epidemiology and clinical manifestations of Adamantiades-Behcet's disease in Germany – current pathogenic concepts and therapeutic possibilities. J Dtsch Dermatol Ges. 2006;4:49–64.
3. Alpsoy E, Zouboulis CC, Ehrlich GE. Mucocutaneous lesions of Behcet's disease. Yonsei Med J. 2007;48:573–85.
4. Ohno S, Ohguchi M, Hirose S, Matsuda H, Wakisaka A, Aizawa M. Close association of HLA-Bw51 with Behcet's disease. Arch Ophthalmol. 1982;100:1455–8.
5. Zouboulis CC, May T. Pathogenesis of Adamantiades-Behcet's disease. Med Microbiol Immunol. 2003;192:149–55.
6. Karaycian A, Zouboulis CC. An update on Behcet's disease. J Eur Acad Dermatol Venereol. 2007;21:1–10.
7. Krause I, Weinberger A. Behcet's disease. Curr Opin Rheumatol. 2008;20:82–7.
8. Kaneko F, Kaneda T, Ohnishi O, Kishiyama K, Takashima I, Fukuda H, Kado Y. Infection allergy in Behcet's disease (1). Jpn J Allergol. 1978;27:440–50.
9. Kaneko F, Oyama N, Nishibu A. Streptococcal infection in the pathogenesis of Behcet's disease and clinical effects of minocycline on the disease symptoms. Yonsei Med J. 1997;38:444–54.
10. Mumcu G, Inanc N, Ergan T, Ikiz K, Gunes M, Islek U, Yavuz S, Sur H, Atalay T, Direskeneli H. Oral health is impaired in Behcet's disease and is associated with disease activity. Rheumatology (Oxford). 2004;43:1028–33.
11. Yokota K, Hayashi S, Araki Y, Isogai E, Kotake S, Yoshikawa K, Fujii N, Hirai Y, Oguma K. Characterization of *Streptococcus sanguinis* isolated from patients with Behcet's disease. Microbiol Immunol. 1995;39:729–32.
12. Isogai E, Ohno S, Takashi K, Yoshikawa K, Turumizu T, Isogai H, Yokota Y, Hashimoto T, Shimizu H, Matsuda H, Fujii N, Yamaguchi M, Oguma K. Close association of *Streptococcus sanguinis* uncommon serotypes with Behcet's disease. Bifidobact Microflora. 1990;9:27–41.
13. Isogai E, Ohno S, Kotake S, Isogai E, Tsurumizu T, Fujii N, Syuto B, Yamaguchi M, Matsuda H, Oguma K. Chemiluminescence of neutrophils from patients with Behcet's disease and its correlation with an increased proportion of uncommon selotypes of *Streptococcus sanguinis* in the oral flora. Arch Oral Biol. 1990;35:43–8.
14. Kaneko F, Takahashi Y, Muramatsu Y, Miura Y. Immunological studies on aphthous ulcer and erythema nodosum-like eruptions in Behcet's disease. Br J Dermatol. 1985;113:303–12.
15. Mizushima Y, Matsuda T, Hoshi K, Ohno S. Induction of Behcet's disease symptoms after dental and streptococcal antigen skin test. J Rheumatol. 1988;15:1029–30.
16. Graykowski EA, Baril MF, Boyd LM, Stanley HR. Recurrent aphthous stomatitis: clinical therapeutic and histopathologic and hypersensitivity aspects. JAMA. 1966;196:637–44.
17. Hirohata S, Oka H, Mizushima Y. Streptococcal antigens stimulate production of IL-6 and interferon-γ by cells from patients with Behcet's disease. Cell Immunol. 1992;140:410–9.
18. Yokota K, Hayashi S, Fujii N, Yoshikawa K, Kotake S, Isogai E, Ohono S, Araki Y, Oguma K. Antibody response to oral streptococci in Behcet's disease. Microbiol Immunol. 1992;36:815–22.
19. Lehner T. The role of heat shock protein, microbial and auto-immune agents in the etiology of Behcet's disease. Int Rev Immunol. 1997;14:21–32.
20. Kaneko S, Suzuki N, Yamashita N, Nagafuchi H, Nakajima T, Wakisaka S, Yamamoto S, Sakane T. Characterization of T cells specific for an epitope of human 60-kD heat shock protein (hsp) in patients with Behcet's disease (BD) in Japan. Clin Exp Immunol. 1997;108:204–12.
21. Kibaroglu A, Eksioglu-Demiralp E, Akoglu T, Direskeneli H. T and NK cell subset changes with microbial extracts and human HSP60-derived peptides in Behcet's disease. Clin Exp Rheumatol. 2004;22 Suppl 34:S59–63.
22. Sakane T, Takeno M, Suzuki N, Inaba G. Current concepts: Behcet's disease. N Engl J Med. 1999;341:1284–91.

23. Suzuki-Krokawa M, Suzuki N. Behcet's disease. Clin Exp Med. 2004;3:10–20.
24. Bang D, Yoon KH, Chung HG, Choi EH, Lee ES, Lee S. Epidemiological and clinical features of Behcet's disease in Korea. Yonsei Med J. 1997;38:428–36.
25. Ship JA. Recurrent aphthous stomatitis. An update. Oral Surg Oral Med Oral Pathol Oral Radiol Oral Endod. 1996;81:141–7.
26. Kaneko F. Behcet's disease. In: Ueki H, Yaoita H, editors. A color atlas of dermato-immunohistology. London: Wolfe Medical Publication; 1989. p. 84–5.
27. Lipschutz B. Ulcer vulvae acutum. In: Jadassohn J, editor. Handbuch der Haut und Geschl, vol. 21. Berlin: Springer; 1927. pp. 392–414.
28. Lee S, Bang D, Lee ES. Behcet's disease. In: The 3rd list of publication on Behcet's disease. 1995–2002, Yonsei University College of Medicine, Seoul, Ajou University School of Medicine, Suwon, Korea; 2003. pp. 27–49.
29. Cho S, Zheng Z, Cho S, Ahn K, Choi M, Kim DY, Lee KH, Bang D. Both the sera of patients with Behcet's disease and Streptococcus sanguinis stimulate membrane expression of hnRNP A2/B1 in endothelial cells. Scand J Rheumatol. 2013;42(3):241–6.
30. Cho SB, Zheng Z, Ahn KJ, Cho S, Kim DY, Lee HS, Bang D. Serum IgA reactivity against GroEL of *Streptococcus sanguinis* and human heterogeneous nuclear ribonucleoprotein A2/B1 in patients with Behcet's disease. Br J Dermatol. 2013;168:977–83.
31. International Study Group for Behcet's Disease. Criteria for diagnosis of Behcet's disease. Lancet. 1990;335:1078–80.
32. Haim S, Sobel JD, Friedman-Brirnbaum R, Liching C. Histological and direct immunofluorescence study of cutaneous hyperreactivity in Behcet's disease. Br J Dermatol. 1976;95:631–5.
33. Jorrizzo JL, Abernothy JL, White WL, Mongelsdorf HC, Zouboulis CC, Sarica R, Gaffney K, Mat C, Yazici H, Al Lalaan A, Assad-Kahalil SH, Kaneko F, Jorizzo EAF. Mucocutaneous criteria for the diagnosis of Behcet's disease: an analysis of clinicopathologic data from multiple international centers. J Am Acad Dermatol. 1995;32:968–76.
34. Srhat-Inaloz H, Evereklioglu C, Unal B, Kirtak N, Eralp A, Inaloz SS. The significance of immunohistochemistry in the skin pathergy reaction of patients with Behcet's syndrome. J Eur Acad Dermatol Venereol. 2004;18:56–61.
35. Davatchi F, Chams-Davachi C, Shahram F, Nadji A, Shams H, Ghodsi Z, Akhlaghi M, Naderi N, Sadechi-Abdolahi B. Pathergy test in Behcet's disease: change in incidence over the time. APLAR J Rheumatol. 2007;10:333–5.
36. Davies PG, Fordham JN, Kirwan JR, Barnes CG, Dinning WJ. The pathergy test and Behcet's syndrome in Britain. Ann Rheum Dis. 1984;43:70–3.
37. Friedman-Birnbaum R, Bergman R, Aizen E. Sensitivity and specificity of pathergy test results in Israeli patients with Behcet's disease. Cutis. 1990;45:261–4.
38. Fresko I, Yazici H, Bayramicli M, Yurdakul S, Mat C. Effect of surgical cleaning of the skin on the pathergy phenomenon in Behcet's syndrome. Ann Rheum Dis. 1993;52:619–20.
39. Togashi A, Saito S, Kaneko F, Nakamura K, Oyama N. Skin prick test with self-saliva in patients with oral aphthosis: A new diagnostic pathergy for Behcet's disease and recurrent aphthosis. Inflamm Allergy Drug Targets. 2011;10:164–70.
40. Kaneko F, Togashi A, Nomura E, Nakamura K. A new diagnostic way for Behcet's disease: Skin prick with self-saliva. Gen Res Intern 2014; http://dx.doi.org/10.1155/2014/581468.
41. Takeno M, Kariyone A, Yamashita N, Takiguchi M, Mizushima Y, Kaneoka H, Sakane T. Excessive function of peripheral blood neutrophils from patients with Behcet's disease and from HLA-B51 transgenic mice. Arthritis Rheum. 1995;38:426–33.
42. Mizuki N, Inoko H, Ohno S. Molecular genetics (HLA) of Behcet's disease. In: Sungnack L, Dongsik B, Eu-So L, Seonghyang S, editors. Behcet's disease: a guide to its clinical understanding. Berlin/New York: Springer; 2001. p. 87–100.
43. Yasuoka H, Okazaki Y, Kawakami Y, Hirakata M, Inoko H, Kuwana M. Autoreactive CD8+ cytotoxic T lymphocytes to major histocompatibility complex class I chain-related gene A in patients with Behcet's disease. Arthritis Rheum. 2004;50:3658–62.

44. Mizuki N, Ota M, Kimura M, Ohno S, Ando H, Katsuyama Y, Yamazaki M, Watanabe K, Goto K, Nakamura S, Bahram S, Inoko H. Triplet repeat polymorphism in the transmembrane region of the MICA gene: a strong association of six GCT repetitions with Behcet's disease. Proc Natl Acad Sci U S A. 1997;94:1298–303.
45. Seo J, Park JS, Nam JH, Bang D, Shon S, Lee ES, Park KS. Association of CD94/NKG2A, CD94/NKG2C and its ligand HLA-E polymorphisms with Behcet's disease. Tissue Antigens. 2007;70:307–13.
46. Kaneko F, Takahashi Y, Muramatsu R, Minagawa T. Natural killer cell numbers and function in peripheral lymphoid cells in Behcet's disease. Br J Dermatol. 1985;113:313–8.
47. Shimizu J, Takai K, Fujiwara N, Arimitsu N, Ueda Y, Wakisaka S, Yoshikawa H, Kaneko F, Suzuki N. Expressive CD4+T cells co-expressing interleukin-17 and interferon-γ in patients with Behcet's disease. Clin Exp Immunol. 2011;168:68–74.
48. Shimizu J, Kaneko F, Suzuki N. Skewed helper T-cell responses to IL-12 family cytokines produced by antigen-presenting cells and the genetic background in Behcet's disease. Gen Res Int. http://dx.doi.org/10.1155/2013/363859
49. Yanagihori H, Oyama N, Nakamura K, Mizuki N, Oguma K, Kaneko F. Role of IL-12B promoter polymorphism in Adamantiades-Behcet's disease susceptibility: An involvement of Th1 immunoreactivity against Streptococcus sanguinis antigen. J Invest Dermatol. 2006;126:1534–40.
50. Isogai E, Isogai H, Kotake S, Ohno Ishihara M, Aeki K, Tojo M, Kaneko F, Yokota K, Oguma K. Antibody cross reactivity from sera of patients with Behcet's disease with synthetic peptides that have homologies with protein from Streptococcus sanguinis. J Appl Res. 2002;2:1–7.
51. Isogai E, Isogai H, Kotake S, Ohno S, Kimura K, Oguma K. Role of *Streptococcus sanguinis* and traumatic factors in Behcet's disease. J Appl Res. 2003;3:64–75.
52. Yoshikawa K, Kotake S, Kubota T, Kimura K, Isogai E, Fujii N. Cloning and sequencing of BES-1 gene encoding the immunogenic antigen of Streptococcus sanguinis KTH-1 isolated from patients with Behcet's disease. Zent bl Bakteriol. 1998;287:449–60.
53. Tojo M, Yanagihori H, Zheng X, Oyama N, Isogai E, Kimura K, Nakamura K, Kaneko F. Bes-1 DNA fragment encoding Streptococcal antigen in skin lesions from patients with Behcet's disease. J Appl Res. 2003;3:232–8.
54. Tojo M, Zheng X, Yanagihori H, Oyama N, Takahashi K, Nakamura K, Kaneko F. Detection of herpes virus genomes in skin lesions from patients with Behcet's disease and other related inflammatory disease. Acta Derm Venereol. 2003;83:1–4.
55. Sohn S, Lee ES, Bang D, Lee S. Behcet's disease-like symptoms induced by the herpes simplex virus in ICR mice. Eur J Dermatol. 1998;8:21–3.
56. Xiang M, Zhou L, Peng Y, Eddy R, Shows TB, Nathans J. Brn 3b: POU domain gene expressed in a subset of retinal ganglion cells. Neuron. 1993;11:689–701.
57. Kulaber A, Tugal-Turkan I, Yentur SP, Akman-Demir G, Kaneko F, Gul A, Saruhan-Direskeneli G. Proinflammatory cellular immune response in Behcet's disease. Rheumatol Int. 2007;27:1113–8.
58. Jindal S, Dudani AK, Singh B, Harley CB, Gupta RS. Primary structure of a human mitochondrial protein homologous to the bacterial and plant chaperonins and to the 65-kilodalton mycobacterial antigen. Mol Cell Biol. 1989;9:2279–83.
59. Lamb JR, Young DB. T cell recognition of stress proteins: a link between infections and autoimmune disease. Mol Biol Med. 1990;7:311–21.
60. Lehner T, Lavery E, Smith R, van der Zee R, Mizushima Y, Shinnick T. Association between the 65-kilodalton heat shock protein, *Streptococcus sanguinis*, and the corresponding antibodies in Behcet's syndrome. Infect Immun. 1991;59:1434–41.
61. Pervin K, Chlderstone A, Shinnick T, Mizushima Y, van der Zee R, Hasan A, Vaughan R, Lehner T. T cell epitope expression of mycobacterial and homologous human 65-kilodalton heat shock protein peptides in short term cell lines from patients with Behcet's disease. J Immunol. 1993;151:2273–82.

62. Poccia F, Pielli P, Vendetti S, Back S, Amendola A, Placido R, Celizzi V. Heat shock protein expression on the membrane of T cells undergoing apoptosis. Immunology. 1996;88:6–12.
63. Ergun T, Ince U, Eksioglu-Demiralp E, Direskeneli H, Gurbuz O, Gurses L, Aker F, Akoglu T. HSP60 expression in mucocutaneous lesions of Behcet's disease. J Am Acad Dermatol. 2001;45:904–9.
64. Direskeneli H, Ekisiogu-Demiralp E, Yavuz S, Ergan T, Shinnick T, Lehner T, Akogl T. T cell responses to 60/65 kDa heat shock protein derived peptides in Turkish patients with Behcet's disease. J Rheumatol. 2000;27:708–13.
65. Imamura Y, Kurokawa MS, Yoshikawa H, Nara K, Takada E, Masuda C, Tsukikawa S, Ozaki S, Matsuda T, Suzuki N. Involvement of Th1 cells and heat shock protein 60 in the pathogenesis of internal Behcet's disease. Clin Exp Immunol. 2005;139:371–8.
66. Direskeneli H. Innate and adaptive responses to heat shock proteins in Behcet's disease. 2013. http://dx.doi.org/10.1155/2013/249157.
67. Direskeneli H, Saruhan-Direskeneli G. The role of heat shock proteins in Behcet's disease. Clin Exp Rheumatol. 2003;21 Suppl 30:S44–8.
68. Shaker O, Ay El-Deen MA, El Hadid H, Grace BD, ElSherif H, Adbel HA. The role of heat shock protein 60, vascular endothelial factor and antiphospholipid antibodies in Behcet's disease. Br J Dermatol. 2007;156:32–7.
69. Yi SW, Kim EH, Kang HY, Kim YC, Lee ES. Erythema nodosum: clinicopathologic correlations and their use in differential diagnosis. Yonsei Med J. 2007;48:601–8.
70. Iikunur T, Pabuccuoglu U, Akin C, Lebe B, Gunes AT. Histopathologic and direct immunofluorescence findings of the papulopustular lesions in Behcet's disease. Eur J Dermatol. 2006;16:146–50.
71. Ates A, Tiryaki OA, Olmez U, Tukkak H. Serum-soluble selectin levels in patients with Behcet's disease. Clin Rheumatol. 2007;26:411–7.
72. Lee MT, Hooper LC, Kump L, Hayashi K, Nussenblatt R, Hooks JJ, Detrick B. Interferon-beta and adhesion molecules (E-selectin and s-intercellular adhesion molecule-1) and detected in sera from patients with retinal vasculitis and are induced in retinal vascular endothelial cells by Toll-like receptor 3 signalling. Clin Exp Immunol. 2007;147:71–80.
73. Yalcin B, Arda N, Tezel GG, et al. Expression of vascular endothelial growth factor and CD34 in oral aphthous lesions of Behcet's disease. Anal Quant Cytol Histol. 2006; 28:303–6.
74. Hu W, Hasan A, Wilson A, Stanford MR, Li-Yang Y, Todryk S, Whiston R, Shinneck T, van der Zee R, Lehner T. Experimental mucosal induction of uveitis with the 60-kDa heat shock protein-derived peptide 336-351. Eur J Immunol. 1998;28:2444–55.
75. Phipps PA, Stanford MR, Sun JB, Xiao BG, Holmgren J, Shinnick T, Hasan A, Mizushima Y, Lehner T. Prevention of mucosally induced uveitis with a HSP60-derived peptide linked to cholera toxin B subunit. Eur J Immunol. 2003;33:224–32.
76. Stanford M, Whittal T, Bergemeier LA, Lindbald M, Lundin S, Shinnick T, Mizushima Y, Holmgren J, Lehner T. Oral tolerization with peptide 336-351 linked to cholera toxin B subunit in preventing relapses of uveitis in Behcet's disease. Clin Exp Immunol. 2004; 137:201–8.
77. Ersoy O, Ersoy R, Yayar O, Demirci H, Tatlican S. H pylori infection in patients with Behcet's disease. World J Gastroenterol. 2007;13:2983–5.
78. Apan TZ, Gursel R, Dolgun A. Increased seropositivity of Helicobacter pylori cytotoxin-associated gene A in Behcet's disease. Clin Rheumatol. 2007;26:88–9.
79. Zouboulis CC, Turnbull JR, Muhlradt F. High seroprevalence of anti-mycoplasma fermentans antibodies in patients with malignant aphthosis. J Invest Dermatol. 2003;121:211–2.
80. Chen ZW, Letvin NL. Adaptive immune response f $V\gamma2V\delta2$ cells: a new paradigm. Trends Immunol. 2003;24:213–9.
81. Bank I, Duvelevani M, Livneh A. Expansion of $\gamma\delta$ T-cells in Behcet's disease: role of disease activity and microbial flora in oral ulcers. J Lab Clin Med. 2003;141:33–41.
82. Radiuddin S, Al-Dalaan A, Bahabri S, Siraj AK, Al-Sedairy S. Divergent cytokine production profile in Behcet's disease. Altered Th1/Th2 cell cytokine pattern. J Rheumatol. 1998; 25:329–33.

83. Hamzaoui K, Hamzaoui A, Ghorbel I, Khanfir M, Houman H. Levels of IL-15 in serum and cerebrospinal fluid of patients with Behcet's disease. Scand J Immunol. 2006;64:655–60.
84. Lew W, Chang JY, Jung TY, Bang D. Increased expression of interleukin-23 p19mRNA in erythema nodosum-like lesion of Behcet's disease. Br J Dermatol. 2008;158:505–11.
85. Zugel U, Kaufman HE. Role of heat shock proteins in protection from and pathogenesis of infectious diseases. Clin Microbiol Rev. 1999;12:19–39.
86. Oguma K, Shin R, Yokota K. Studies on immunological responses by bacterial antigens in Behcet's disease. Report of the Research Group for Behcet's disease organized by the Japanese Ministry of Health, Labour and Welfare 2006–2007; 2008. pp. 31–3 (in Japanese).
87. Kaneko F, Togashi A, Nomura E, Nakamura K, Isogai E, Yokota K, Oguma K. Role of heat shock protein derived from Streptococcus sanguinis in Behcet's disease. J Med Microbiol Diagn. 2012;S.2. http://dx.doi.org/10.4172/2161-0703.S2-001
88. Zarember KA, Godowski PJ. Tissue expression of human Toll-like receptors and differential regulation of Toll-like receptor mRNAs in leukocytes in response to microbes, their products, and cytokines. J Immunol. 2002;168:554–61.
89. Hornung V, Rothenfusser S, Britsch S, Krug A, Jahrsdörfer B, Giese T, Endres S, Hartmann G. Quantitative expression of Toll-like receptor 1-10 mRNA in cellular subsets of human peripheral blood mononuclear cells and sensitivity to CpG oligodeoxynucleotides. J Immunol. 2002;168:4531–7.
90. Yavus S, Elbir Y, Tulunay A, Eksioglu-Demirap E, Direskeneli H. Differential expression of toll-like receptor 6 on granulocytes and monocytes implicates the role of microorganisms in Behcet's disease etiopathogenesis. Rheumatol Int. 2007. doi:10.1007/s00296-007-0470-y.
91. Durranni O, Wallace GR, Hamburger J, et al. Toll-like receptors (TLRs) expression in oral ulcer biopsies from Behcet's disease (BD) patients: a role for the innate immune system in BD. Clin Exp Rheumatol. 2004;22 Suppl 34:S1–93.
92. Medzhitov R, Janeway CA. Innate immunity. N Engl J Med. 2000;343:338–44.
93. Kilpatrick DC. Mannose-binding lectin: clinical significance and applications. Biochim Biophys Acta. 2002;1572:401–13.
94. Inanc N, Mumcu G, Birtas E, Blsir Y, Yavuz S, Fresko I, Direskeneli H. Serum mannose-binding lectin levels are decreased in Behcet's disease and associated with disease severity. J Rheumatol. 2005;32:287–91.
95. Matsushita M, Fujita T. The role of ficolins in innate immunity. Immunobiology. 2002; 205:490–7.
96. Lynch NJ, Roscher S, Hartung T, Morath S, Matsushita M, Maennel DN, Kuraya M, Fujita T, Schwaeble WJ. L-ficolin specifically binds to lipoteic acid, a cell wall constituent of Gram-positive bacteria and activates the lectin pathway of complement. J Immunol. 2004;172:1198–202.
97. Wang H, Nakamura K, Inoue T, Yanagihori H, Kawakami Y, Hashimoto S, Oyama N, Kaneko F, Fujita T, Nishida T, Mizuki N. Mannose-binding lectin polymorphisms in patients with Behcet's disease. J Dermatol Sci. 2004;36:115–7.
98. Chen X, Katoh Y, Nakamura K, Oyama N, Kaneko F, Endo Y, Fujita T, Nishida T, Mizuki N. Single nucleotide polymorphisms of Ficolin 2 gene in Behcet's disease. J Dermatol Sci. 2006;43:201–5.
99. Calguneri M, Ertenli I, Kiraz S, Ertenli I, Benek-Li M, Karaarslan Y, Celik I. Effect of prophylactic benzathine penicillin on mucocutaneous symptoms of Behcet's disease. Dermatology. 1996;192:125–8.
100. Mumcu G, Inac N, Yavuz S, Direskeneli H. The role of infectious agents in the pathogenesis, clinical manifestations and treatment strategies in Behcet's disease. Clin Exp Rheumatol. 2007;25:S27–33.
101. Kaneko F, Oyama N, Yanagihori H, Isogai E, Yokota K, Oguma K. The role of streptococcal hypersensitivity in the pathogenesis of Behcet's disease. Eur J Dermatol. 2008;18:489–98.
102. Kaneko F, Togashi A, Saito S, Sakuma H, Oyama N, Nakamura K, Yokota K, Oguma K. Behcet's disease (Adamantiades-Behcet's disease). Clin Dev Immunol 2011; ID 681956: 7 page. doi:10.1155/2011/681956.

Chapter 9
Perspective

Yoshiaki Ishigatsubo and Mitsuhiro Takeno

Abstract We review four cases of Behçet's disease patients with serious organ involvement. Case 1 developed an aneurysm in the left subclavian artery, which was successfully treated with emergent endovascular intervention followed by infliximab. Case 2 repeated acute neurological attacks during infliximab therapy for pre-existing ocular involvement. Sustained elevation of IL-6 in cerebrospinal fluid suggested transition to chronic progressive type of neuro-Behçet's disease. Cases 3 and 4 had surgical operations for intestinal perforation of ileocecal ulcers. Case 3 needed reoperation for anastomotic leakage, while Case 4 had a third operation in spite of treatment with infliximab and adalimumab after second operation. We have learned both potent efficacy and limitation of anti-TNF therapy for BD patients.

Lastly, we would like to show our trial to establish an animal model with disease susceptible genes which have been identified by genome-wide association study and subsequent investigation, leading to a novel therapeutic strategy for more appropriate targets in Behçet's disease.

Keywords Vasculo-Behçet's disease • Neuro-Behçet's disease • Intestinal Behçet's disease • Infliximab • HLA-B51 • ERAP-1

9.1 Introduction

Recent progression in each topic of Behçet's disease (BD) is described in previous chapters. Based on the accumulated findings, we have to consider the next step. The European League Against Rheumatism (EULAR) recommendations summarize the therapeutic approaches for different aspects of BD [1]. However, some patients are still suffering from the disease despite application of therapeutic options in addition to standard therapies.

Y. Ishigatsubo, M.D., Ph.D. (✉) • M. Takeno
Department of Internal Medicine and Clinical Immunology, Yokohama City University Graduate School of Medicine, 3-9 Fukuura, Kanazawa-Ku, Yokohama 236-0004, Japan
e-mail: ishigats@med.yokohama-cu.ac.jp

Y. Ishigatsubo (ed.), *Behçet's Disease*,
DOI 10.1007/978-4-431-54487-6_9

We have learned a lot from patients. In this chapter, four case presentations are shown based on our experience over the last 5 years. All cases occurred after 2007 approval of infliximab (IFX) for ocular lesions. Thus, available therapeutic options are equivalent to those at present.

9.2 Lessons from Patients with Serious Organ Involvement

9.2.1 Subclavian Artery Aneurysm Treated with Infliximab After Endovascular Intervention

Case 1 A 41-year-old male patient visited a neighborhood clinic because of fever, pseudofolliculitis of the legs, and right hip arthralgia. He was referred to our department because vasculitis was suspected. Symptoms spontaneously subsided without any therapy prior to diagnosis (Fig. 9.1).

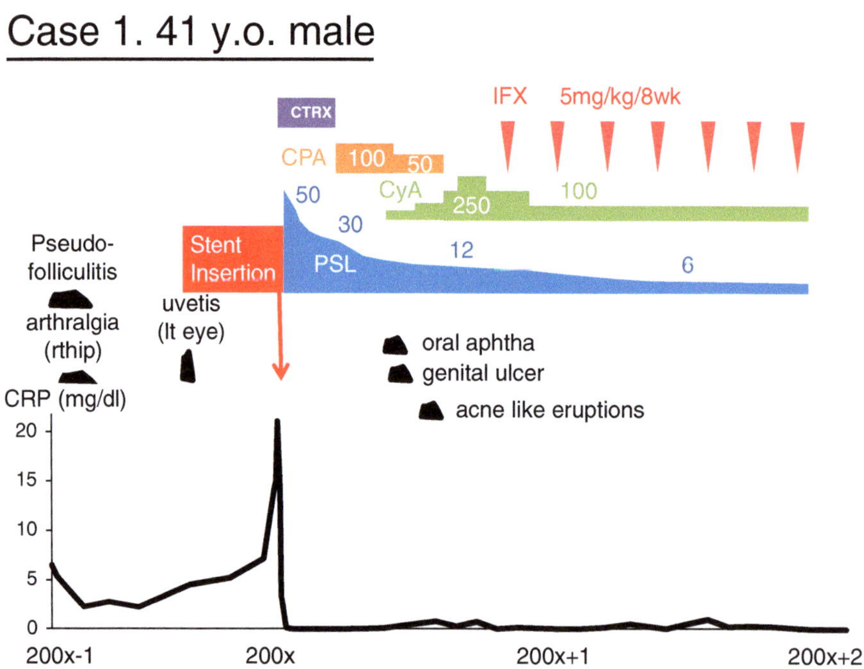

Fig. 9.1 Clinical course of Case 1 (41-year-old male) with subclavian artery aneurysm. Endovascular intervention followed by corticosteroid relieved vascular symptoms, but ocular and mucocutaneous symptoms developed in spite of concomitant immunosuppressants. Eleven months later, infliximab (IFX) suppression was started, resulting in remission. *CTRX* ceftriaxone, *CPA* cyclophosphamide, *CyA* cyclosporine A, *PSL* prednisolone

He had been well 1 year later until he presented with sudden onset of blurred vision in the left eye, which was diagnosed as uveitis at a neighborhood ophthalmology clinic, though the underlying disease remained undetermined. Another 3 months later, he was admitted to our department because a painful and pulsating tumor was growing in the left cervical region. On physical examination, there was no abnormality except low-grade fever (37.3 °C), difference in blood pressure between the right arm (118/78 mmHg) and the left (98/62 mmHg), and bruit on the left cervical tumor. Laboratory data showed leukocytosis (14,800/mm^3) and increased CRP (14.1 mg/dl). Autoantibodies including rheumatoid factor, antinuclear antibody (ANA), proteinase-3-antineutrophil cytoplasmic antibody (ANCA), and myeloperoxidase-ANCA were all negative. Blood culture did not detect any pathogens. HLA typing revealed A24 and A26, but HLA-B was undetermined. Of note, HLA-A26 is a susceptible genetic marker for BD in Japanese population [2, 3].

Contrast-enhanced and three-dimensional CT scans demonstrated pseudoaneurysm with a 7 cm diameter in the left subclavian artery at the distal portion of branching of the vertebral artery (Fig. 9.2a, b). The portion corresponded to a

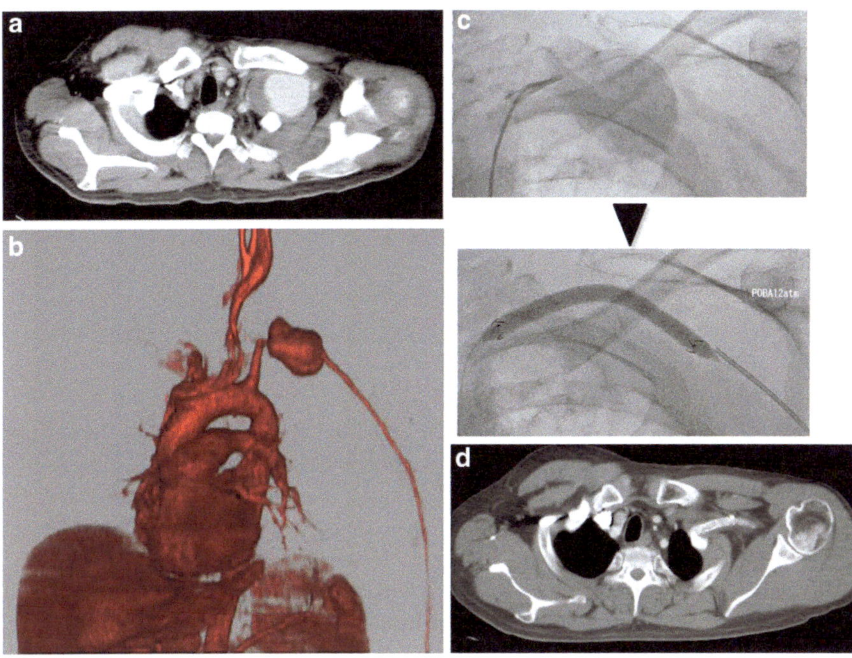

Fig. 9.2 CT findings of pseudoaneurysm in the left subclavian artery of Case 1. (**a**) Contrast-enhanced CT scan showed a mass lesion with 7 cm of diameter in the left subclavian artery. Vascular wall thickness in the distal portion of the aneurysm suggests arteritis. (**b**) Three-dimensional CT illustrated aneurysm in the left subclavian artery. (**c**) A cover was inserted into the aneurysm lesion by endovascular intervention, leading to sufficient blood flow to the left upper limb. (**d**) A follow-up CT scan showed diminished size of the aneurysm with a diameter of 4 cm and a good blood flow through the stent

pulsating tumor on the body surface in physical examinations. Vascular wall thickening in the distal portion of the pseudoaneurysm suggested inflammatory aneurysm. Surgical operation was suspended, because differential diagnosis included infectious aneurysm and vasculo-BD. At this point, the diagnosis of BD can be made according to the Japan revised criteria [4] (Chap. 1, Table 1.5), though the patient did not meet the diagnostic criteria of the International Study Group (ISG criteria) (Chap. 1, Table 1.3), because of the lack of oral aphthosis [5]. Instead of surgical resection, 50 mg/day of PSL and ceftriaxone were initiated immediately after admission. On the evening of admission, severe left shoulder pain suddenly developed, suggesting impending aneurysm rupture. A cover stent was inserted into the lesion via emergency endovascular intervention (Fig. 9.2c), leading to sufficient blood flow to the left arm and reduction of the pressure to the aneurysm wall. Thereafter, symptoms subsided with normalization of laboratory data. He was discharged 40 days after hospitalization and followed in the outpatient clinic. During tapering of prednisolone, mucocutaneous symptoms such as oral aphthosis, genital ulcers, and acne-like eruptions became apparent with slight elevation of CRP level, in spite of treatment with PSL and cyclophosphamide. Switching from cyclophosphamide to cyclosporine A was also ineffective. IFX was initiated 11 months later after endovascular therapy, resulting in remission without major relapse of vascular events. A follow-up CT scan revealed that the aneurysm size had diminished to 4 cm diameter and that the inserted stent remained patent with sufficient blood flow to the left upper limb (Fig. 9.2d).

This case has at least two important messages in treatment and diagnosis. Endovascular therapy was selected in this case instead of surgical operation which is often associated with postoperative complications and relapses [6–15]. As discussed in Table 5.3 of Chap. 5, previous reports have suggested that mortality, recurrence, and occlusion are less frequent in endovascular therapy than surgical operation, though direct comparison is difficult among the studies [7–13, 15–19]. Immunosuppressive therapy is associated with favorable outcomes in BD patients with vascular involvement, though there is no firm evidence to guide the management of major vessel disease in BD [1, 20–22]. Concomitant preoperative immunosuppressive therapies have also shown to reduce postoperative complications [7, 23]. In this case, no vascular event developed after starting IFX, which was originally used for ocular involvement. Sporadic case reports have shown beneficial effects of TNF inhibitors on vascular involvement [24] (see Sect. 5.7.4). In Japan, IFX is now under clinical trial for BD patients with vascular involvement. This case suggests that endovascular treatment with TNF inhibitors can be a promising option in impending rupture of peripheral artery aneurysms, instead of surgery with conventional immunosuppressive therapies.

Another issue is diagnosis, as discussed in Chap. 1. The patient had not met ISG criteria until oral aphthosis appeared 3 months after the episode of impending aneurysm rupture. However, the diagnosis could be made at the episode according to the Japan revised criteria and the International Criteria for Behçet's Disease (ICBD) (see Chap. 1, Tables 1.3, 1.4, 1.5) [25]. Both sets of criteria are more sensitive than the ISG criteria, because vascular and neurological lesions are taken into account. Early diagnosis based on the sensitive criteria is critical when patients have life-threatening symptoms like this case.

The Japan Behçet's Disease Research Committee is now generating "Recommendations for management of vasculo-Behçet's Disease based on consensus in Japan." The draft is shown in Appendix 9.1.

9.2.2 Relapsing Acute Episodes of Neuro-Behçet's Disease During Infliximab Therapy for Preexisting Uveitis

Case 2 A 29-year-old female patient was diagnosed with BD based on oral aphthosis, erythema nodosum-like eruptions on the left leg, and genital ulcer 3 months ago. Because ocular attacks in the left eye developed in spite of colchicine treatment, she was referred to our department where IFX was started at 6 months after the diagnosis. Although ocular attacks were suppressed, she often experienced transient headaches. Because of oral herpes, the six courses of IFX administration were suspended. One week later, she presented with high fever (39.3 °C), oral aphthoid ulcers, acne-like eruptions on the cheeks, erythema nodosum on the legs, and severe headache. Laboratory data showed leukocytosis (10,100/mm^3) and a slightly elevated CRP level (0.41 mg/dl). HLA typing revealed A22, A31, B7, and B51. Cerebrospinal fluid examination showed pleocytosis (1,432/3 mm^3) and elevated protein (136 mg/dl) with remarkably increased IL-6 8,620 pg/ml and glucose at 54 mg/dl. CSF culture was negative. Emergency MRI demonstrated sporadic high intensity signals on T2-weighted image/FLAIR in the left thalamus, cerebral white matter, left middle cerebellar peduncle, and cerebellar hemisphere (Fig. 9.4). Based on these findings, the diagnosis of acute neuro-BD was made. The findings were also compatible with preliminary diagnostic criteria for the classification of acute neuro-BD proposed by the Japan Behçet's Disease Research Committee (Chap. 6, Table 2) [26]. She received steroid pulse therapy (methyl PSL 1,000 mg/day × 3 days) followed by 30 mg/day of oral PSL. In response to corticosteroids, clinical manifestations subsided with drastic reduction of IL-6 and cell numbers in CSF within 2 weeks (Fig. 9.3). The follow-up MRI revealed that T2 signals disappeared in the thalamus and cerebellum. However, IL-6 level was increased again and cell numbers remained above 100/3 μl 1 month later, after the neurological attack. The abnormal findings continued. Four months later, she had severe headache recurrence. Mucocutaneous symptoms of BD also repeated despite treatment with IFX and weekly methotrexate. Eventually, she was rehospitalized due to another neurological attack, which was treated with high dose PSL.

Treatment for neuro-BD is summarized in Sect. 6.5. Corticosteroid therapy is the first line for acute neurological attacks, but the effects are short lived and they do not prevent recurrence of attacks [27]. This was true for the aforementioned case. The

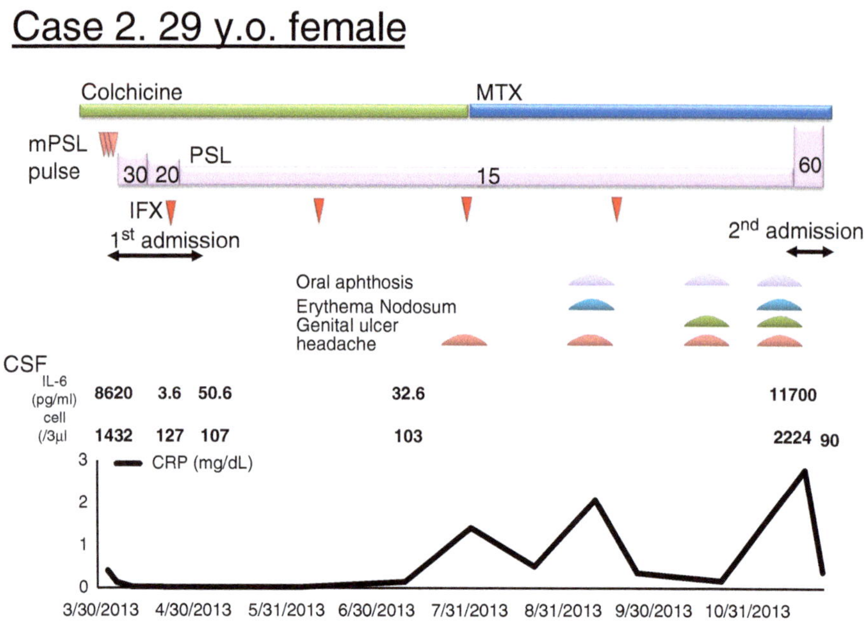

Fig. 9.3 Clinical course of Case 2 (29-year-old male) with repeated acute neurological attacks during treatment with infliximab. Steroid pulse therapy showed a transient reduction of CSF IL-6 levels with the improvement of clinical manifestations. In spite of restart of infliximab, mucocutaneous symptoms and headache recurred

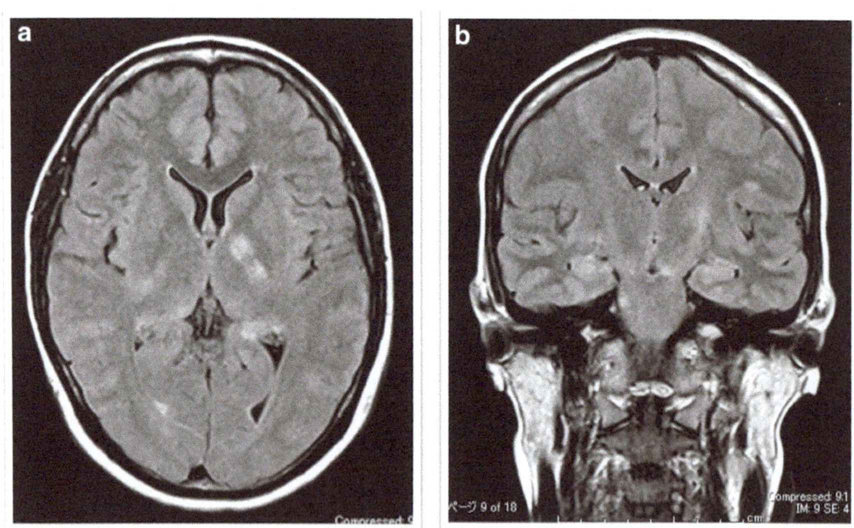

Fig. 9.4 MRI findings at the first acute neurological attack in Case 2. (**a**) Axial view and (**b**) frontal view. Sporadic high-intensity signals were found in the left thalamus, cerebral white matter, left middle cerebellar peduncle, and cerebellar hemisphere on T2-weighted image/FLAIR

first acute neurological attacks responded well to corticosteroids including pulse therapy, but she repeated another episode despite colchicine administration, which was shown to have preventive effects on relapsing acute neurological attacks by a retrospective Japan multicenter cohort study [28].

CSF findings remained abnormal in the patient even after subsiding manifestations of the first acute episode. Particularly, IL-6 in CSF, a possible biomarker in chronic progressive neuro-BD, had been elevated persistently, suggesting chronic neurological involvement (see Chap. 6) [26, 29, 30]. Most of immunosuppressive therapies including corticosteroids are little effective in the type of neuro-BD [29, 31, 32], whereas MTX and/or IFX show beneficial effects in some of the patients, but not all [33–35]. The efficacy is associated with normalization of CSF IL-6 level [34, 35]. In this case, however, suppressive effects of MTX and IFX on CSF IL-6 level appeared insufficient. Fortunately, she has not yet presented the other characteristic features for chronic progressive neuro-BD, such as progressive brainstem atrophy in MRI and clinical features including dementia/neurobehavior changes, ataxia, and dysarthria [26, 36], at least until the last observation. Careful monitoring of MRI as well as CSF is also important in the future.

9.2.3 Intestinal Perforation in Two Intestinal BD Patients

Case 3 A 64-year-old male patient was admitted to our department because of high fever and massive melena. He had been diagnosed with BD since he was 50 years old, when he had oral aphthosis, genital ulcer, pseudofolliculitis, and polyarthritis. Treatment with colchicine and weekly MTX were initiated. He presented with mild uveitis 5 years ago. Colonoscopy showed punched-out ulcer in the terminal ileum (Fig. 9.5a) when he was referred to our hospital 3 years ago. PSL (25 mg/day) and mesalazine were started in addition to colchicine and MTX, but the ulcer enlarged without responding to the therapies. TNF inhibitors were proposed as alternative treatment, but clinical trial of adalimumab was suspended because screening chest CT scan detected a nodular shadow which was suspicious of lung cancer, though it spontaneously disappeared. A year later, he was admitted to our hospital due to fever (38 °C) and massive melena after he had been suffering from right lower abdominal pain, anorexia, general malaise, and diarrhea for a month. Physical examinations on admission revealed hypotension (BP 73/48 mmHg) with tachycardia (PR 123 bpm) and local tenderness and defense in the right lower abdomen. Laboratory data showed progressive anemia (Hb 9.9 g/dal) and elevated CRP levels. Contrast-enhanced CT scans demonstrated peritoneal abscess around the ileocecal region (Fig. 9.5b), leading to the diagnosis of peritonitis due to perforation of the ileocecal region and septic shock. He received emergency ileocecectomy, confirming perforation sites. A week later, reoperation was conducted because of anastomotic leak. After the second operation, abdominal symptoms were controlled with low doses of PSL, MTX, mesalazine, and colchicine.

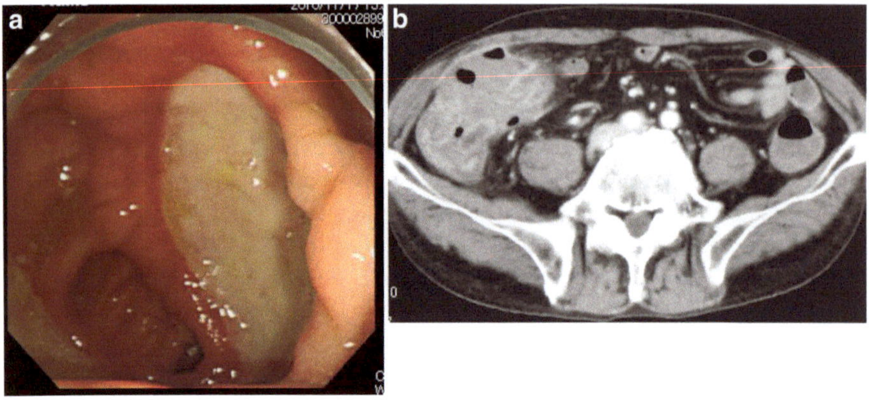

Fig. 9.5 Ileocecal ulcer and development of abscess in Case 3. (**a**) Endoscopic examination revealed a giant punched-out ulcer in the terminal ileum. The findings had not been improved for more than a year in spite of PSL, MTX, mesalazine, and colchicine. (**b**) Contrast-enhanced CT findings showed mixed densities and air in the enlarged ileocecal region suggesting abscess before the emergency operation

Case 4 A 44-year-old female patient was admitted to our department for IFX initiation for intestinal BD, because she had already surgical laparotomy twice for intestinal perforation at 13 and 43 years old. The diagnosis of BD had been made during her first operation when she presented with oral aphthosis, genital ulcers, and erythema nodosum. Postoperative therapies including PSL and salazosulfapyridine successfully induced remission. Thereafter, she had been well for 30 years until a second perforated ileum resection. One year later, IFX was initiated due to active intestinal ulcers with stenosis remaining in the terminal ileum despite treatment with PSL, mesalazine, and weekly MTX. However, obstructive ileus developed after the 5th administration with IFX (Fig. 9.6). The ileus was resolved by methyl PSL pulse therapy, but switching from MTX to cyclosporine A (CyA) and trial of adalimumab were unsuccessful as a maintenance therapy. One year later, she had another episode of intestinal perforation, requiring a third ileocecectomy. In the resected specimen, multiple ulcers were found including the terminal ileum perforation site (Fig. 9.7). After initiating tacrolimus, PSL was gradually tapered without major intestinal exacerbations until the last observation.

Intestinal lesions are more frequently found in BD patients from Far East Asian countries such as Korea and Japan than from other areas (Chap. 7, Table 7.1) [37]. In EULAR recommendations, the statement for intestinal lesion is as follows [1]: "There is no evidence-based treatment that can be recommended for the management of gastrointestinal involvement of BD. Agents such as sulfasalazine, corticosteroids, azathioprine, TNF-α antagonists and thalidomide should be tried first before surgery, except in emergencies." Detail therapeutic strategies are discussed in Sect. 7.7.

Both Case 3 and Case 4 required multiple surgical operations because of perforation of the terminal ileum, with the highest prevalence of intestinal lesions in

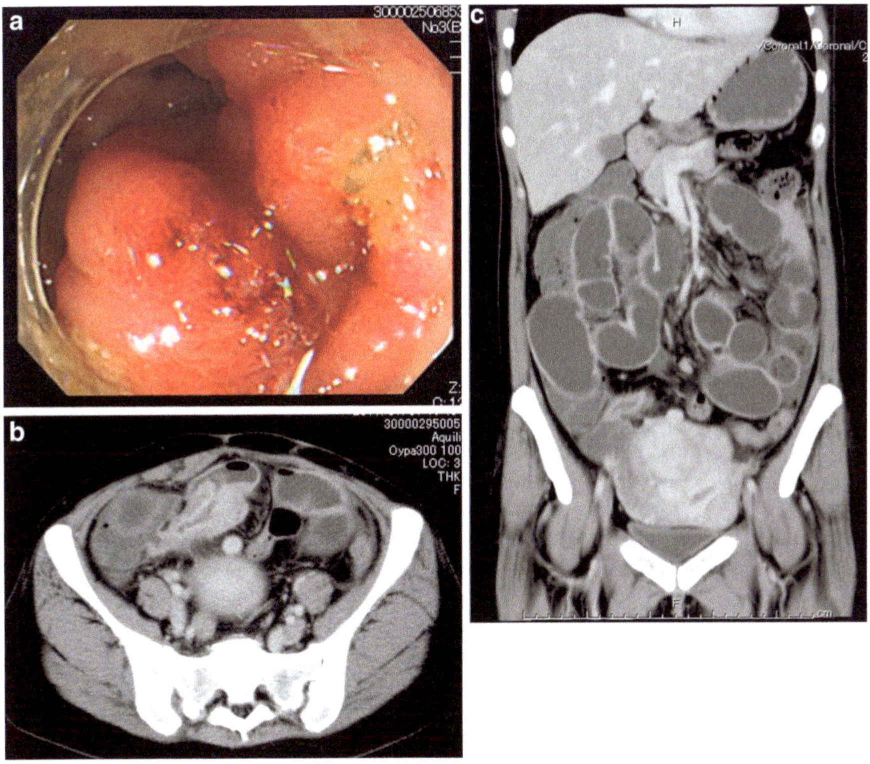

Fig. 9.6 Ileocecal ulcer and development of ileus in Case 4. (**a**) Endoscopic examination revealed ileocecal ulcer with stenosis. (**b**, **c**) Contrast-enhanced CT findings showed thickness of terminal ileum wall with contrast effects, leading to the local stenosis. Fluid retention in the proximal small intestine indicated obstructive ileus

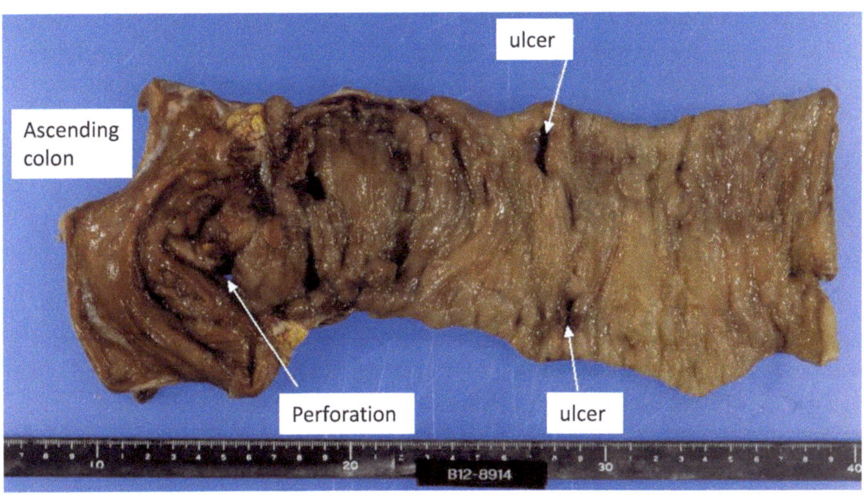

Fig. 9.7 Resected ileocecal region in the third operation in Case 4. Multiple ulcers and scars were found including the perforating site of the terminal ileum

BD. However, both the patients had different backgrounds. In Case 3, insufficient therapy may be responsible for the development of intestinal perforation, because TNF inhibitors were suspended. On the other hand, Case 4 was refractory to available pharmacological therapies including two kinds of anti-TNF mAb, resulting in intestinal perforation which required the third operation.

Reports from Korea and Japan have shown that perforation of the ileocecal ulcer is the leading cause of surgical operations [38–41], as described here in the two cases. Surgical treatment is not always associated with favorable clinical outcomes, due to frequency of postoperative complications and recurrences. Based on these data, operative indication is restricted in emergency or patients having refractory intestinal lesions to conservative therapies. Postoperative complications include anastomotic leak, local infection, and GI bleeding (Table 9.1). Recurrence is the most frequent in the anastomosis site. Mechanical suture using a stapler should be avoided because local pathergy-like reaction may be involved in local recurrence and anastomotic leak.

Predisposing factors to intestinal perforation and operation in BD patients include young-aged onset, failure of early remission induction by pharmacological therapies, punched-out or volcano-shaped ulcers, and history of previous operations [39, 40]. Concurrent pharmacological therapy is also related with complications and recurrence. Recurrence rate is significantly reduced in patients receiving azathioprine [39]. On the other hand, postoperative steroid therapy is associated with high frequency of reoperation such as in Case 3 [41]. Although immunosuppression plays a principle role in treatment for BD, it seems important to minimize steroid dose in the management of patients with intestinal BD, especially those with a surgical history. Although we have not reached consensus concerning indication of TNF antagonists, a previous survey in Japan revealed that around 40 % of intestinal BD patients receiving IFX had a history of previous operations (unpublished observation). Indeed, Iwata et al. have shown that IFX revealed a significant steroid-sparing effect in addition to potent efficacy for intestinal involvement [42, 43].

"Consensus statements for the diagnosis and management of intestinal Behçet's disease (second edition)," by Research Committee for small bowel inflammation of unknown etiology and Behçet's Disease Research Committee, Ministry of Health, Labour, and Welfare, Japan, is shown in Appendix 9.2 [44].

9.3 Efficacy and Limitation of TNF Antagonists for BD

A number of studies have shown that anti-TNFα therapy has greatly contributed to the improvement of clinical outcomes in BD patients, irrespective of the subtypes. In all of 4 patients discussed here, treatment with anti-TNFα mAb was tried or considered because of refractory organ involvement. However, the indication of the TNF inhibitors for BD patients is determined by different criteria among institutes and physicians. Moreover, some patients are suffering from serious organ involvement which is refractory to TNF inhibitors, like Case 2 and Case 4. These cases suggest limitation of TNF antagonists in the treatment of BD.

Table 9.1 Surgical operation and the outcomes in intestinal BD patients

		Total patients	Operation		Intestinal perforation	Ileocecal lesions	Postoperative complication	Recurrence	Recurrence in the anastomosis	Reoperation
		N	*N*	/Total patients	/Operation	/Perforation	/Operation	/Operation	/Recurrence	/Operation
Kasahara Y,	1981	–	136	–	56 %	76 %	44 % Re-perforation anastomotic leak, suture failure, sepsis, GI bleeding	40 %	Almost	44 %
Choi IJ,	2000	43	22	51 %	52 %	NA	NA	2 years 49 % 5 years 75 %	81 %	55 %
Moon CM	2010	129	33	26 %	100 %	52 %	Local infection 5, GI bleeding 2, death (sepsis) 1	42 %	86 %	33 %
Jung YS,	2011	–	72	–	58 %	86 %	GI bleeding 2 Enterocutaneous fistula 2	58 %	93 %	31 %

NA not available

Clinical observation in BD patients receiving IFX for uveitis has raised another issue in the treatment. Discontinuation of IFX is frequently accompanied by recurrence of ocular attacks in BD patients with refractory uveitis [45]. Our preliminary study in BD patients with uveitis shows that the efficacy of IFX depends on the serum trough level and that ocular attacks repeat with shortage of the agent in the body. It is hard to discontinue the therapy or to determine when it can be discontinued safely even in patients with a favorable clinical course under treatment with IFX. This is in contrast to interferon-α, which shows a long-lasting effect after the cessation [46]. It is likely that TNF inhibitors suppress amplified immune responses mediated by TNF, but do not directly correct the underlying immune abnormality in BD. The absence of susceptible genes in the TNF signaling pathway also suggests that excessive TNF synthesis might play a secondary role in the pathophysiology of the disease. Agents with distinct mode of actions might be considered for clinical application to intractable conditions in BD.

9.4 Reconstruction of Immunogenetic Findings; To Elucidate the Pathogenesis

It is important to elucidate the pathogenesis of BD at molecular levels for the development of novel therapeutic strategies. There is accumulating evidence that both genetic and environmental factors are implicated in the development of BD, but most of the recent studies have focused on the genetics.

After a strong association of HL-A5 with BD was first reported in 1973 [47], a number of subsequent studies from different ethnic groups have shown that HLA-B51 is the most important genetic predisposition to BD [48]. On the other hand, case–control studies using candidate-gene approaches have suggested some candidates of non-HLA susceptible genes in BD patients, but most of them were not replicated in different ethnic groups. In 2010, gene-wide association studies (GWAS) identified *IL10* and *IL12RB-IL23R* as susceptible genes besides *HLA* in two independent patient populations, Japan and Turkey [3, 49]. It is of note that the data were replicated in other ethnic populations which almost covered the prevalent areas of BD, indicating that the findings are universal. A series of subsequent studies have further identified susceptible genes, most of which are related with the innate and acquired immune systems [50–52]. Details are discussed in Sect. 9.3.

We are now in the post-genomic era. It is necessary to confirm the function of the identified susceptible genes in the patients and to reconstruct the pathophysiology based on the findings. The processes are essential to consider the next therapeutic strategies. *HLA-B51* is the first identified and the most specific genetic preposition to BD, whereas other susceptible genes are shared with other inflammatory disorders. However, the role of HLA-B51 remains uncertain, though implication in disease-specific antigen presentation to CD8+ T cells has been suggested [53, 54]. Kirino et al. recently identified *ERAP1* as a novel susceptible gene encoding endoplasmic reticulum aminopeptidase 1 (ERAP1) which trims proteasome-derived peptides from their amino terminals before being loaded onto the antigen-binding groove of HLA class I molecules [50]. Interestingly, the risk *ERAP1* variants preferentially confer risk for BD in *HLA-B*51*-positive individuals. The epistasis of the *ERAP1* variants with HLA class I genes is also found in *HLA-B*27*-positive ankylosing spondylitis individuals [55] and *HLA-C*06*-positive psoriasis individuals [56], though the risk *ERAP1* allele confers protection of ankylosing spondylitis and psoriasis. It is likely that the *ERAP1* variants determine repertoire of antigenic peptides which are presented by HLA class I molecules, resulting in the disease-specific immune responses.

Mizuki et al., our collaborators, are now generating third-generation *HLA-B*51* transgenic mice which express HLA-B51 linking with human β2-microglobulin in the absence of murine MHC class I. Furthermore, the *ERAP1* risk or protective allele knock-in mice are also being generated. The genetically modified mice may contribute to understanding the pathogenesis of BD, leading to the development of a novel therapeutic strategy.

9.5 Summary

Biologics, particularly TNF inhibitors, have contributed to the improvement of clinical outcomes in many BD patients, but some patients are still suffering from serious conditions which are resistant to currently available therapies. Recent advances in immunogenetics in this field shed new light on the pathogenesis of BD.

Appendices

Appendix 9.1: Draft – "Recommendations for Management of Vasculo-Behçet's Disease Based on Consensus in Japan, 2014"

Purposes

Vascular involvement can be lethal and one of the most critical manifestations in patients with Behçet's disease. The statements are mainly focused on Japanese patients, based on literatures and a retrospective cohort study conducted in 105 patients with vasculo-Behçet's disease by Behçet's Disease Research Committee, Ministry of Health, Labour, and Welfare, Japan.

I.	Conception and epidemiology in Japan		
	(1)	*Definition*	
		The diagnosis of vascular type of Behçet's disease or vasculo-Behçet's disease is made according to the Japan criteria. The patients must meet complete or incomplete type of the criteria. The statements are not applicable or may be only suggestive for probable cases of Behçet's disease.	
		The presence of vascular lesions is confirmed by clinical findings and imaging modalities. Superficial thrombophlebitis belongs to one of the skin symptoms according to the Japan criteria, but it is of note that the lesions are frequently accompanied by deep vessel lesions.	
	(2)	*Epidemiology*	
		Previous studies, which surveyed 277 to 3,316 patients with Behçet's disease in Japan, have shown that vascular involvement is found in 6.3–15.3 % of the patients. Serious form of vascular lesions is more common in young-aged male than female.	
		In the survey of Research Committee, vascular lesions are distributed as follows: the venous lesions 71. 4 % (thrombosis 68.6 %), the arterial lesions 29.5 % (aneurysm 19.0 %, occlusion 12.4 %), pulmonary lesions 24.8 % (pulmonary thrombosis 19.0 %, aneurysm 7.6 %), and cardiac lesions 6.7 %. The data were consistent with previous reports from various countries. The coexistence of multiple lesions and recurrences is common, as shown in the survey of the Research Committee, which detected multiple lesions in 46.7 % and recurrences in 24.8 % of the patients. Arterial lesions, especially pulmonary lesions, are frequently accompanied by venous lesions. Bleeding from pulmonary artery, aneurysm rupture, and cardiac lesions can be lethal.	
		In the survey of the Research Committee, vascular manifestations were found at the diagnosis in 25.7 % and preceded to the diagnosis in 1.9 % of the patients. Mean duration from the diagnosis of Behçet's disease to the onset of vascular manifestations was 7.1 ± 7.9 years.	
	(3)	*Pathology*	
		(a)	Venous system: Inflammation of the venous wall is involved in obstructive thrombosis.
		(b)	Arterial system: Neutrophils and lymphocytes infiltrate into the media to adventitia of arterial wall followed by fibrotic changes. The obstruction of *vasa vasorum* causes necrosis of the arterial wall, resulting in aneurysm formation.
		(c)	Pulmonary circulatory system: Mononuclear cells dominantly infiltrate into *vasa vasorum* of the pulmonary artery, leading to aneurysm and thrombosis in situ. Pulmonary embolism is rare despite of frequent complication of deep vein thrombosis. However, some disagree with the statement.

(continued)

II.	Clinical symptoms and diagnostic procedures		
	(1)	*Clinical symptoms*	
		Vascular lesions are often multiple and recurrent, as shown in the epidemiology. When a vascular lesion is found, another lesion should be surveyed and monitored.	
		(a)	Venous lesion: Deep vein thrombosis is the most frequent in the lower limbs, but it also occurs in the superior vena cava, inferior vena cava, hepatic vein, and cerebral sinus. The lesions lead to peripheral edema distal to thrombosis, dilatation of superficial veins as collateral circulation, and skin ulcers. Superior and inferior vena cava syndrome and Budd–Chiari syndrome have been reported. Cerebral sinus thrombosis causes non-parenchymal type of neuro-Behçet's disease, but it is rare in Japan.
		(b)	Arterial lesion: Arterial involvement is associated with systemic symptoms such as fever and general malaise in acute phase. Arterial occlusion is responsible for ischemic symptoms in the territory. Aneurysm is prevalent in large-sized artery including aorta and the pulmonary artery. Peripheral aneurysm is often palpable as pulsating tumor with tenderness on the body surface, whereas intra-abdominal aneurysm may grow asymptomatically until rupture leads to lethal bleeding.
		(c)	Pulmonary lesion: Pulmonary vascular lesions cause cough, chest pain, dyspnea, and hemoptysis.
		(d)	Cardiac lesion: Although the frequency is rare, valvular disease, especially aortic regurgitation, endomyocardial fibrosis, coronary angiitis, endocardial thrombosis, and conducting disorders have been reported.
	(2)	*Imaging findings*	
		Imaging modalities including intravenous digital subtraction angiography (IVDSA), contrast-enhanced CT scan, three-dimensional (3D) CT scan, MRI/MRA, and pulmonary perfusion scintigraphy are useful to detect vascular lesions. FDG-PET/CT scan evaluates the activity of inflammatory lesion in addition to anatomical localization.	
		The following modalities are used for individual lesions:	
		(a)	Venous lesion: ultrasonography, contrast-enhanced CT scan, and MRI/MRA.
		(b)	Arterial lesion: ultrasonography, contrast-enhanced CT scan, 3D CT scan, MRI/MRA, and IVDSA. Direct puncture of artery should be avoided except therapeutic endovascular intervention, because the procedure has a risk to induce the puncture site aneurysm.
		(c)	Pulmonary vessels: spiral CT, 3D CT, CT angiography, MRA, and FDG-PET/CT.
		(d)	Cardiac lesion: ultrasound cardiography (UCG), coronary CT, MRI, and myocardial scintigraphy. It is important to assess function in addition to morphological evaluation.
	(3)	*Laboratory examinations*	
		(a)	Hematological examinations: Although there is no disease-specific biomarker, D-dimer and inflammatory findings such as ESR and CRP are supportive indicators.
		(b)	Genetic factor: No genetic predisposition to vasculo-Behçet's disease has been identified.
	(4)	*Differential diagnosis*	
		(a)	Venous lesion: Thrombosis due to idiopathic vein thromboembolism, coagulopathy such as protein C and protein S deficiency, antiphospholipid antibody syndrome, surgical stress, malignancy, and mechanical compression should be excluded.
		(b)	Arterial lesion: Inflammatory aneurysm due to aortitis syndrome, infected aneurysm, periarteritis nodosum, and arterial occlusion due to Buerger disease and arteriosclerosis obliterans are considered as differential diagnoses.
		(c)	Pulmonary vessels: Hemoptysis caused by infectious diseases such as tuberculosis, especially during immunosuppressive therapy, is taken into account.
	(5)	*Assessment of disease activity*	
		Disease activity is comprehensively assessed by clinical manifestations, laboratory data, and imaging findings.	

(continued)

III.	Treatment			
	(1)	*Therapeutic goal in vasculo-Behçet's disease is to avoid lethal events which related with rupture of aneurysm and pulmonary bleeding and to relieve various symptoms caused by vascular involvement.*		
	(2)	*Pharmacological therapy*		
		(a)	Immunosuppressive therapy: Corticosteroids and immunosuppressants have shown to be effective for active vascular lesions, irrespective of arterial and venous lesions. Early treatment is recommended with careful screening and monitoring of latent infections such as tuberculosis, hepatitis B virus, and hepatitis C virus.	
			(i)	Corticosteroids with concomitant immunosuppressants are used for acute phase of aneurysm and pulmonary artery involvement. Starting dose of oral prednisolone (PSL, 0.5–1 mg/kg/day) is continued 2–4 weeks followed by tapering the dose under careful monitoring. Pulse therapy (methyl prednisolone 1,000 mg/day × 3 days) is considered in serious cases. Concomitant immunosuppressive therapies include intravenous cyclophosphamide (IVCY), which is administered along the regimens for vasculitis syndrome or lupus nephritis, weekly methotrexate, azathioprine, and cyclosporine.
			(ii)	Treatment with azathioprine, cyclophosphamide, or cyclosporine A suppresses development and recurrence of thrombophlebitis and deep vein thrombosis.
			(iii)	The efficacy of anticoagulant in addition to immunosuppressants and colchicine has been shown for cardiac lesions.
		(b)	Biologics: Sporadic case reports have suggested that biologics, particularly TNF inhibitors, are promising options for vasculo-Behçet's disease.	
		(c)	Anticoagulant treatment: Anticoagulants, antiplatelets, or antifibrinolytic agents should be avoided in patients with pulmonary vascular lesions, especially pulmonary artery aneurysms, which have a high risk of fatal hemoptysis. On the other hand, reports from France, the UK, and Japan have shown that pulmonary bleeding is not common even in patients receiving anticoagulants and antiplatelets for venous thrombosis and arterial lesions, respectively.	
			Beneficial effects of anticoagulants have been shown on intracardiac thrombosis, myocardial infarction, and cerebral sinus thrombosis.	
	(3)	*Surgical operation*		
		Impending rupture of aneurysm and active bleeding from vascular lesions require emergency operation. Otherwise, immunosuppressive therapies should be tried first before surgery, because recurrences and postoperative complications such as aneurysm formation at the anastomosis site are frequent. Pre- and postoperative concurrent immunosuppressive therapies are associated with favorable outcomes of surgical operation.		
	(4)	*Endovascular treatment*		
		Endovascular intervention can be alternatives for operation in some cases under concomitant immunosuppressive therapies, because the local recurrence of aneurysm has been reported after the procedure.		
	(5)	*Prevention of recurrence*		
		Recurrence is less common in patients receiving immunosuppressive therapy. Anticoagulant therapy is helpful for the prevention of graft occlusion.		
	(6)	*Therapy for extravascular lesions*		
		Therapies for coexistent lesions including ocular involvement should be arranged with individual specialists.		

Appendix 9.2

"Consensus statements for the diagnosis and management of intestinal Behçet's disease (second edition)," by Research Committee for small bowel inflammation of unknown etiology and Behçet's Disease Research Committee, Ministry of Health, Labour, and Welfare, Japan (Hisamatsu et al. [44])

<table>
<tr><td colspan="3">Concept of the second edition of consensus statements</td></tr>
<tr><td colspan="3">According to the increased use of anti-TNFα mAb in inflammatory bowel disease, many cases of intestinal Behçet's disease in which anti-TNFα mAb (infliximab, IFX) showed efficacy also have been reported in Japan. The same tendency was observed in foreign countries that have a high prevalence of Behçet's disease, such as Korea. In 2013, adalimumab, humanized anti-TNFα mAb, was approved for intestinal Behçet's disease in Japan. In the second edition, statements have focused on where we should place anti-TNFα mAb for the treatment of intestinal Behçet's disease based on relevant literature and expert panel discussion[a]</td></tr>
<tr><td colspan="3">Diagnosis</td></tr>
<tr><td>(1)</td><td colspan="2">Diagnosis of intestinal Behçet's disease can be made if</td></tr>
<tr><td></td><td>(A)</td><td>There is a typical oval-shaped large ulcer in the terminal ileum, OR</td></tr>
<tr><td></td><td>(B)</td><td>There are ulcerations or inflammation in the small or large intestine, and clinical findings meet the diagnostic criteria of Behçet's disease[b]</td></tr>
<tr><td>(2)</td><td colspan="2">Acute appendicitis, infectious enteritis, tuberculosis, Crohn's disease, nonspecific colitis, drug-associated colitis, and other diseases that mimic intestinal Behçet's diseases should be excluded by clinical findings, radiology, and endoscopy before diagnosis of intestinal Behçet's disease is made</td></tr>
<tr><td colspan="3">Assessment of severity</td></tr>
<tr><td colspan="3">Disease severity should be comprehensively assessed by systemic symptoms (e.g., fever, extraintestinal manifestations), physical examinations of abdomen (e.g., pain, inflammatory mass, rebound tenderness), depth of ulcers and intestinal complications (e.g., bleeding, stricture, fistula), inflammatory mediators (e.g., CRP, WBC, ESR), and anemia</td></tr>
<tr><td colspan="3">Treatment objectives</td></tr>
<tr><td colspan="3">In the treatment of intestinal Behçet's disease, as well as the improvement of abdominal and extraintestinal symptoms, the achievement of negative levels of CRP could be desirable. In the long-term prognosis, the prevention of progression to disability and poly-surgery is important</td></tr>
<tr><td>(A)</td><td colspan="2">Standard treatment</td></tr>
<tr><td></td><td>(1)</td><td>In patients with severe symptoms (i.e., abdominal pain, diarrhea, gastrointestinal bleeding) and complications with deep ulcers confirmed by radiology or endoscopy, corticosteroids should be considered for induction therapy. The initial dose of corticosteroids is 0.5–1 mg/kg per day of prednisolone for 1–2 weeks. When clinical improvement is observed, prednisolone should be tapered by 5 mg every week and finally stopped. ADA (approved on May 16, 2013 in Japan) could be considered for induction therapy [160 mg at 0 w, 80 mg at 2 w, 40 mg at 4 w, subcutaneously (s.c.)]. In responders, scheduled maintenance therapy should be considered (40 mg s.c. every other week). IFX (not approved yet) could also be considered for induction therapy (5 mg/kg at week 0, 2, and 6). In responders, scheduled maintenance therapy every 8 weeks should be considered. In patients with mild to moderate activity, mesalamine (5-ASA) could be effective for induction therapy. In patients treated with corticosteroids, anti-TNFα mAbs, and immunomodulators, infectious disease and neoplasm should be surveyed. After initiation of these therapies, the risk of infectious disease and neoplasm should be monitored continuously</td></tr>
</table>

(continued)

	(2)	In patients who are induced to clinical remission, 5-ASA and colchicine could be used for maintenance therapy. The optimal dose of 5-ASA for adult patients is 2.25–3 g/day. When sulfasalazine (SASP) is used, the optimal dose is 3–4 g/day
	(3)	[c]Immunosuppressive agents such as azathioprine (AZA)c are indicated when patients are corticosteroid dependent, corticosteroid resistant, or anti-TNFα mAb resistant. The initial dose of AZA is 25–50 mg/day. In patients treated with AZA, adverse effects (e.g., neutropenia and liver dysfunction) should be monitored
	(4)	Total parenteral nutrition (TPN) is indicated for patients with severe systemic symptoms such as fever and for patients with intestinal complications such as stenosis, fistula, bleeding, and impending perforation. TPN is also indicated for patients who cannot orally intake drugs due to severe oral or upper gastrointestinal lesions. It is usually used for a limited period of time considering the risk of catheter infection and thrombosis. After the patient's condition is improved by TPN, enteral nutrition (EN) could be considered
	(5)	EN using an elementary diet could be effective for induction therapy. It is indicated in particular for patients with refractory disease, severe activity, and disability such as stricture lesions. When EN is introduced, adherence and quality of life of the patients should be considered
	(6)	Surgery is indicated for patients in whom improvement is not expected by medications. Patients with severe stricture lesions, perforations, large abscesses, and massive gastrointestinal bleedings have an absolute indication. Patients refractory to medications, and with a low quality of life due to intestinal complications such as fistula, have a relative indication of surgery. Minimum length of resection surgery should be considered
	(7)	The risk of postoperative recurrence is high in patients with volcano-shaped deep ulcers and fistulas. Postoperative recurrence often occurs at anastomosis. Although a treatment strategy has not been established that can reduce the risk of postoperative recurrence, considering the high risk of postoperative recurrence and poly-surgeries, medication by 5-ASA, immunomodulators, metronidazole, anti-TNFα mAb, and EN could be considered for postoperative management
	(8)	In patients with intestinal Behçet's disease complicated with eye lesions, consultation with ophthalmologists is necessary for their management
(B)	Optional treatment	
	Since there are some case reports showing that spraying of absolute ethanol via endoscope has efficacy for ulcers of intestinal Behçet's disease, it could be considered in refractory patients	
	Expecting the efficacy as an antirheumatoid arthritis drug, change from 5-ASA to SASP could be considered in patients with arthritis (especially peripheral arthritis)	

The authors state that (1) most of the consensus statements are based on expert opinions, (2) the consensus statements have not been endorsed by any organizations, (3) the consensus statements need to be prospectively reevaluated, (4) the consensus statements do not cover histopathological diagnosis, and (5) the consensus statements do not have any binding force

[a]The majority of literature regarding anti-TNFα therapy in intestinal Behçet's disease that is referred to for the establishment of the second edition described the efficacy of infliximab. On May 16, 2013, ADA was approved for intestinal Behçet's disease. The clinical trial of infliximab in intestinal Behçet's disease is currently in progress in Japan

[b]Diagnosis of Behçet's disease is according to the Japanese criteria proposed in 2003

[c]Immunomodulators besides AZA, including 6-mercaptopurine, cyclosporine, tacrolimus, and methotrexate, could be considered, but consultations with specialists who have sufficient experience are required. When considering the use of these drugs, adverse effects should be monitored

References

1. Hatemi G, Silman A, Bang D, Bodaghi B, Chamberlain AM, Gul A, Houman MH, Kotter I, Olivieri I, Salvarani C, Sfikakis PP, Siva A, Stanford MR, Stubiger N, Yurdakul S, Yazici H, Committee EE. EULAR recommendations for the management of Behcet disease. Ann Rheum Dis. 2008;67(12):1656–62. doi:10.1136/ard.2007.080432.
2. Mizuki N, Ohno S, Ando H, Chen L, Palimeris GD, Stavropoulos-Ghiokas E, Ishihara M, Goto K, Nakamura S, Shindo Y, Isobe K, Ito N, Inoko H. A strong association between HLA-B*5101 and Behcet's disease in Greek patients. Tissue Antigens. 1997;50(1):57–60.
3. Mizuki N, Meguro A, Ota M, Ohno S, Shiota T, Kawagoe T, Ito N, Kera J, Okada E, Yatsu K, Song YW, Lee EB, Kitaichi N, Namba K, Horie Y, Takeno M, Sugita S, Mochizuki M, Bahram S, Ishigatsubo Y, Inoko H. Genome-wide association studies identify IL23R-IL12RB2 and IL10 as Behcet's disease susceptibility loci. Nat Genet. 2010;42(8):703–6. doi:10.1038/ng.624.
4. Ideguchi H, Suda A, Takeno M, Ueda A, Ohno S, Ishigatsubo Y. Behcet disease: evolution of clinical manifestations. Medicine. 2011;90(2):125–32. doi:10.1097/MD.0b013e318211bf28.
5. International Study Group for Behcet's Disease. Criteria for diagnosis of Behcet's disease. Lancet. 1990;335(8697):1078–80.
6. Le Thi HD, Wechsler B, Papo T, Piette JC, Bletry O, Vitoux JM, Kieffer E, Godeau P. Arterial lesions in Behcet's disease. A study in 25 patients. J Rheumatol. 1995;22(11):2103–13.
7. Park MC, Hong BK, Kwon HM, Hong YS. Surgical outcomes and risk factors for postoperative complications in patients with Behcet's disease. Clin Rheumatol. 2007;26(9):1475–80. doi:10.1007/s10067-006-0530-9.
8. Tuzun H, Besirli K, Sayin A, Vural FS, Hamuryudan V, Hizli N, Yurdakul S, Yazici H. Management of aneurysms in Behcet's syndrome: an analysis of 24 patients. Surgery. 1997;121(2):150–6.
9. Nitecki SS, Ofer A, Karram T, Schwartz H, Engel A, Hoffman A. Abdominal aortic aneurysm in Behcet's disease: new treatment options for an old and challenging problem. Isr Med Assoc J. 2004;6(3):152–5.
10. Hosaka A, Miyata T, Shigematsu H, Shigematsu K, Okamoto H, Ishii S, Miyahara T, Yamamoto K, Akagi D, Nagayoshi M, Nagawa H. Long-term outcome after surgical treatment of arterial lesions in Behcet disease. J Vasc Surg. 2005;42(1):116–21. doi:10.1016/j.jvs.2005.03.019.
11. Kalko Y, Basaran M, Aydin U, Kafa U, Basaranoglu G, Yasar T. The surgical treatment of arterial aneurysms in Behcet disease: a report of 16 patients. J Vasc Surg. 2005;42(4):673–7. doi:10.1016/j.jvs.2005.05.057.
12. Iscan ZH, Vural KM, Bayazit M. Compelling nature of arterial manifestations in Behcet disease. J Vasc Surg. 2005;41(1):53–8. doi:10.1016/j.jvs.2004.09.018.
13. Koksoy C, Gyedu A, Alacayir I, Bengisun U, Uncu H, Anadol E. Surgical treatment of peripheral aneurysms in patients with Behcet's disease. Eur J Vasc Endovasc Surg. 2011;42(4):525–30. doi:10.1016/j.ejvs.2011.05.010.
14. Tuzun H, Seyahi E, Arslan C, Hamuryudan V, Besirli K, Yazici H. Management and prognosis of nonpulmonary large arterial disease in patients with Behcet disease. J Vasc Surg. 2012;55(1):157–63. doi:10.1016/j.jvs.2011.07.049.
15. Yang SS, Park KM, Park YJ, Kim YW, Do YS, Park HS, Park KB, Kim DI. Peripheral arterial involvement in Behcet's disease: an analysis of the results from a Korean referral center. Rheumatol Int. 2013;33(8):2101–8. doi:10.1007/s00296-013-2700-9.
16. Okada K, Eishi K, Takamoto S, Ando M, Kosakai Y, Nakano K, Sasako Y, Kobayashi J. Surgical management of Behcet's aortitis: a report of eight patients. Ann Thorac Surg. 1997;64(1):116–9.
17. Kwon TW, Park SJ, Kim HK, Yoon HK, Kim GE, Yu B. Surgical treatment result of abdominal aortic aneurysm in Behcet's disease. Eur J Vasc Endovasc Surg. 2008;35(2):173–80. doi:10.1016/j.ejvs.2007.08.013.

18. Kim WH, Choi D, Kim JS, Ko YG, Jang Y, Shim WH. Effectiveness and safety of endovascular aneurysm treatment in patients with vasculo-Behcet disease. J Endovasc Ther. 2009;16(5):631–6. doi:10.1583/09-2812.1.
19. Liu CW, Ye W, Liu B, Zeng R, Wu W, Dake MD. Endovascular treatment of aortic pseudoaneurysm in Behcet disease. J Vasc Surg. 2009;50(5):1025–30. doi:10.1016/j.jvs.2009.06.009.
20. Hatemi G, Silman A, Bang D, Bodaghi B, Chamberlain AM, Gul A, Houman MH, Kotter I, Olivieri I, Salvarani C, Sfikakis PP, Siva A, Stanford MR, Stubiger N, Yurdakul S, Yazici H. Management of Behcet disease: a systematic literature review for the European League Against Rheumatism evidence-based recommendations for the management of Behcet disease. Ann Rheum Dis. 2009;68(10):1528–34. doi:10.1136/ard.2008.087957.
21. Saadoun D, Asli B, Wechsler B, Houman H, Geri G, Desseaux K, Piette JC, du Huong LT, Amoura Z, Salem TB, Cluzel P, Koskas F, Resche-Rigon M, Cacoub P. Long-term outcome of arterial lesions in Behcet disease: a series of 101 patients. Medicine. 2012;91(1):18–24. doi:10.1097/MD.0b013e3182428126.
22. Desbois AC, Wechsler B, Resche-Rigon M, Piette JC, Huong Dle T, Amoura Z, Koskas F, Desseaux K, Cacoub P, Saadoun D. Immunosuppressants reduce venous thrombosis relapse in Behcet's disease. Arthritis Rheum. 2012;64(8):2753–60. doi:10.1002/art.34450.
23. Ha YJ, Jung SY, Lee KH, Jung SJ, Lee SW, Park MC, Lee SK, Shim WH, Chang BC, Park YB. Long-term clinical outcomes and risk factors for the occurrence of post-operative complications after cardiovascular surgery in patients with Behcet's disease. Clin Exp Rheumatol. 2012;30(3 Suppl 72):S18–26.
24. Adler S, Baumgartner I, Villiger PM. Behcet's disease: successful treatment with infliximab in 7 patients with severe vascular manifestations. A retrospective analysis. Arthritis Care Res. 2012;64(4):607–11. doi:10.1002/acr.21557.
25. International Team for the Revision of the International Criteria for Behcet's D. The International Criteria for Behcet's Disease (ICBD): a collaborative study of 27 countries on the sensitivity and specificity of the new criteria. J Eur Acade Dermatol Venereol. 2014;28(3):338–47. doi:10.1111/jdv.12107.
26. Hirohata S, Kikuchi H, Sawada T, Nagafuchi H, Kuwana M, Takeno M, Ishigatsubo Y. Clinical characteristics of neuro-Behcet's disease in Japan: a multicenter retrospective analysis. Mod Rheumatol. 2012;22(3):405–13. doi:10.1007/s10165-011-0533-5.
27. Al-Araji A, Kidd DP. Neuro-Behcet's disease: epidemiology, clinical characteristics, and management. Lancet Neurol. 2009;8(2):192–204. doi:10.1016/s1474-4422(09)70015-8.
28. Hirohata S, Kikuchi H, Sawada T, Nagafuchi H, Kuwana M, Takeno M, Ishigatsubo Y. Analysis of various factors on the relapse of acute neurological attacks in Behcet's disease. Mod Rheumatol. 2014. doi:10.3109/14397595.2014.891496.
29. Hirohata S, Isshi K, Oguchi H, Ohse T, Haraoka H, Takeuchi A, Hashimoto T. Cerebrospinal fluid interleukin-6 in progressive Neuro-Behcet's syndrome. Clin Immunol Immunopathol. 1997;82(1):12–7.
30. Hirohata S, Kikuchi H. Changes in biomarkers focused on differences in disease course or treatment in patients with neuro-Behcet's disease. Intern Med. 2012;51(24):3359–65.
31. Akman-Demir G, Serdaroglu P, Tasci B, The Neuro-Behcet Study Group. Clinical patterns of neurological involvement in Behcet's disease: evaluation of 200 patients. Brain. 1999;122(Pt 11):2171–82.
32. Siva A, Altintas A, Saip S. Behcet's syndrome and the nervous system. Curr Opin Neurol. 2004;17(3):347–57.
33. Kikuchi H, Aramaki K, Hirohata S. Low dose MTX for progressive neuro-Behcet's disease. A follow-up study for 4 years. Adv Exp Med Biol. 2003;528:575–8. doi:10.1007/0-306-48382-3_117.
34. Kikuchi H, Aramaki K, Hirohata S. Effect of infliximab in progressive neuro-Behcet's syndrome. J Neurol Sci. 2008;272(1–2):99–105. doi:10.1016/j.jns.2008.05.002.
35. Hirohata S, Suda H, Hashimoto T. Low-dose weekly methotrexate for progressive neuropsychiatric manifestations in Behcet's disease. J Neurol Sci. 1998;159(2):181–5.

36. Kikuchi H, Takayama M, Hirohata S. Quantitative analysis of brainstem atrophy on magnetic resonance imaging in chronic progressive neuro-Behcet's disease. J Neurol Sci. 2014;337(1–2):80–5. doi:10.1016/j.jns.2013.11.020.
37. Davatchi F, Shahram F, Chams-Davatchi C, Shams H, Nadji A, Akhlaghi M, Faezi T, Ghodsi Z, Faridar A, Ashofteh F, Sadeghi Abdollahi B. Behcet's disease: from East to West. Clin Rheumatol. 2010;29(8):823–33. doi:10.1007/s10067-010-1430-6.
38. Kasahara Y, Tanaka S, Nishino M, Umemura H, Shiraha S, Kuyama T. Intestinal involvement in Behcet's disease: review of 136 surgical cases in the Japanese literature. Dis Colon Rectum. 1981;24(2):103–6.
39. Choi IJ, Kim JS, Cha SD, Jung HC, Park JG, Song IS, Kim CY. Long-term clinical course and prognostic factors in intestinal Behcet's disease. Dis Colon Rectum. 2000;43(5):692–700.
40. Moon CM, Cheon JH, Shin JK, Jeon SM, Bok HJ, Lee JH, Park JJ, Hong SP, Kim TI, Kim NK, Kim WH. Prediction of free bowel perforation in patients with intestinal Behcet's disease using clinical and colonoscopic findings. Dig Dis Sci. 2010;55(10):2904–11. doi:10.1007/s10620-009-1095-7.
41. Jung YS, Yoon JY, Lee JH, Jeon SM, Hong SP, Kim TI, Kim WH, Cheon JH. Prognostic factors and long-term clinical outcomes for surgical patients with intestinal Behcet's disease. Inflamm Bowel Dis. 2011;17(7):1594–602. doi:10.1002/ibd.21517.
42. Iwata S, Saito K, Yamaoka K, Tsujimura S, Nawata M, Hanami K, Tanaka Y. Efficacy of combination therapy of anti-TNF-alpha antibody infliximab and methotrexate in refractory entero-Behcet's disease. Mod Rheumatol. 2011;21(2):184–91. doi:10.1007/s10165-010-0370-y.
43. Iwata S, Saito K, Yamaoka K, Tsujimura S, Nawata M, Suzuki K, Tanaka Y. Effects of anti-TNF-alpha antibody infliximab in refractory entero-Behcet's disease. Rheumatology. 2009;48(8):1012–3. doi:10.1093/rheumatology/kep126.
44. Hisamatsu T, Ueno F, Matsumoto T, Kobayashi K, Koganei K, Kunisaki R, Hirai F, Nagahori M, Matsushita M, Kobayashi K, Kishimoto M, Takeno M, Tanaka M, Inoue N, Hibi T. The 2nd edition of consensus statements for the diagnosis and management of intestinal Behcet's disease: indication of anti-TNF alpha monoclonal antibodies. J Gastroenterol. 2014;49(1):156–62. doi:10.1007/s00535-013-0872-4.
45. Ohno S, Nakamura S, Hori S, Shimakawa M, Kawashima H, Mochizuki M, Sugita S, Ueno S, Yoshizaki K, Inaba G. Efficacy, safety, and pharmacokinetics of multiple administration of infliximab in Behcet's disease with refractory uveoretinitis. J Rheumatol. 2004;31(7):1362–8.
46. Deuter CM, Zierhut M, Mohle A, Vonthein R, Stobiger N, Kotter I. Long-term remission after cessation of interferon-alpha treatment in patients with severe uveitis due to Behcet's disease. Arthritis Rheum. 2010;62(9):2796–805. doi:10.1002/art.27581.
47. Ono S, Aoki K, Sugiura S, Nakayama E, Itakura K. Letter: HL-A5 and Behcet's disease. Lancet. 1973;2(7842):1383–4.
48. Gul A. Genetics of Behcet's disease: lessons learned from genomewide association studies. Curr Opin Rheumatol. 2014;26(1):56–63. doi:10.1097/bor.0000000000000003.
49. Remmers EF, Cosan F, Kirino Y, Ombrello MJ, Abaci N, Satorius C, Le JM, Yang B, Korman BD, Cakiris A, Aglar O, Emrence Z, Azakli H, Ustek D, Tugal-Tutkun I, Akman-Demir G, Chen W, Amos CI, Dizon MB, Kose AA, Azizlerli G, Erer B, Brand OJ, Kaklamani VG, Kaklamanis P, Ben-Chetrit E, Stanford M, Fortune F, Ghabra M, Ollier WE, Cho YH, Bang D, O'Shea J, Wallace GR, Gadina M, Kastner DL, Gul A. Genome-wide association study identifies variants in the MHC class I, IL10, and IL23R-IL12RB2 regions associated with Behcet's disease. Nat Genet. 2010;42(8):698–702. doi:10.1038/ng.625.
50. Kirino Y, Bertsias G, Ishigatsubo Y, Mizuki N, Tugal-Tutkun I, Seyahi E, Ozyazgan Y, Sacli FS, Erer B, Inoko H, Emrence Z, Cakar A, Abaci N, Ustek D, Satorius C, Ueda A, Takeno M, Kim Y, Wood GM, Ombrello MJ, Meguro A, Gul A, Remmers EF, Kastner DL. Genome-wide association analysis identifies new susceptibility loci for Behcet's disease and epistasis between HLA-B*51 and ERAP1. Nat Genet. 2013;45(2):202–7. doi:10.1038/ng.2520.

51. Kirino Y, Zhou Q, Ishigatsubo Y, Mizuki N, Tugal-Tutkun I, Seyahi E, Ozyazgan Y, Ugurlu S, Erer B, Abaci N, Ustek D, Meguro A, Ueda A, Takeno M, Inoko H, Ombrello MJ, Satorius CL, Maskeri B, Mullikin JC, Sun HW, Gutierrez-Cruz G, Kim Y, Wilson AF, Kastner DL, Gul A, Remmers EF. Targeted resequencing implicates the familial Mediterranean fever gene MEFV and the toll-like receptor 4 gene TLR4 in Behcet disease. Proc Natl Acad Sci U S A. 2013;110(20):8134–9. doi:10.1073/pnas.1306352110.
52. Ombrello MJ, Kirino Y, de Bakker PI, Gul A, Kastner DL, Remmers EF. Behcet disease-associated MHC class I residues implicate antigen binding and regulation of cell-mediated cytotoxicity. Proc Natl Acad Sci U S A. 2014. doi:10.1073/pnas.1406575111.
53. Yasuoka H, Okazaki Y, Kawakami Y, Hirakata M, Inoko H, Ikeda Y, Kuwana M. Autoreactive CD8+ cytotoxic T lymphocytes to major histocompatibility complex class I chain-related gene A in patients with Behcet's disease. Arthritis Rheum. 2004;50(11):3658–62. doi:10.1002/art.20597.
54. Yasuoka H, Yamaguchi Y, Mizuki N, Nishida T, Kawakami Y, Kuwana M. Preferential activation of circulating CD8+ and gammadelta T cells in patients with active Behcet's disease and HLA-B51. Clin Exp Rheumatol. 2008;26(4 Suppl 50):S59–63.
55. Evans DM, Spencer CC, Pointon JJ, Su Z, Harvey D, Kochan G, Oppermann U, Dilthey A, Pirinen M, Stone MA, Appleton L, Moutsianas L, Leslie S, Wordsworth T, Kenna TJ, Karaderi T, Thomas GP, Ward MM, Weisman MH, Farrar C, Bradbury LA, Danoy P, Inman RD, Maksymowych W, Gladman D, Rahman P, Morgan A, Marzo-Ortega H, Bowness P, Gaffney K, Gaston JS, Smith M, Bruges-Armas J, Couto AR, Sorrentino R, Paladini F, Ferreira MA, Xu H, Liu Y, Jiang L, Lopez-Larrea C, Diaz-Pena R, Lopez-Vazquez A, Zayats T, Band G, Bellenguez C, Blackburn H, Blackwell JM, Bramon E, Bumpstead SJ, Casas JP, Corvin A, Craddock N, Deloukas P, Dronov S, Duncanson A, Edkins S, Freeman C, Gillman M, Gray E, Gwilliam R, Hammond N, Hunt SE, Jankowski J, Jayakumar A, Langford C, Liddle J, Markus HS, Mathew CG, McCann OT, McCarthy MI, Palmer CN, Peltonen L, Plomin R, Potter SC, Rautanen A, Ravindrarajah R, Ricketts M, Samani N, Sawcer SJ, Strange A, Trembath RC, Viswanathan AC, Waller M, Weston P, Whittaker P, Widaa S, Wood NW, McVean G, Reveille JD, Wordsworth BP, Brown MA, Donnelly P. Interaction between ERAP1 and HLA-B27 in ankylosing spondylitis implicates peptide handling in the mechanism for HLA-B27 in disease susceptibility. Nat Genet. 2011;43(8):761–7. doi:10.1038/ng.873.
56. Strange A, Capon F, Spencer CC, Knight J, Weale ME, Allen MH, Barton A, Band G, Bellenguez C, Bergboer JG, Blackwell JM, Bramon E, Bumpstead SJ, Casas JP, Cork MJ, Corvin A, Deloukas P, Dilthey A, Duncanson A, Edkins S, Estivill X, Fitzgerald O, Freeman C, Giardina E, Gray E, Hofer A, Huffmeier U, Hunt SE, Irvine AD, Jankowski J, Kirby B, Langford C, Lascorz J, Leman J, Leslie S, Mallbris L, Markus HS, Mathew CG, McLean WH, McManus R, Mossner R, Moutsianas L, Naluai AT, Nestle FO, Novelli G, Onoufriadis A, Palmer CN, Perricone C, Pirinen M, Plomin R, Potter SC, Pujol RM, Rautanen A, Riveira-Munoz E, Ryan AW, Salmhofer W, Samuelsson L, Sawcer SJ, Schalkwijk J, Smith CH, Stahle M, Su Z, Tazi-Ahnini R, Traupe H, Viswanathan AC, Warren RB, Weger W, Wolk K, Wood N, Worthington J, Young HS, Zeeuwen PL, Hayday A, Burden AD, Griffiths CE, Kere J, Reis A, McVean G, Evans DM, Brown MA, Barker JN, Peltonen L, Donnelly P, Trembath RC. A genome-wide association study identifies new psoriasis susceptibility loci and an interaction between HLA-C and ERAP1. Nat Genet. 2010;42(11):985–90. doi:10.1038/ng.694.

Index

Y. Ishigatsubo (ed.), *Behçet's Disease*,
DOI 10.1007/978-4-431-54487-6

V

MIX
Papier aus verantwortungsvollen Quellen
Paper from responsible sources
FSC® C105338

If you have any concerns about our products,
you can contact us on
ProductSafety@springernature.com

In case Publisher is established outside the EU,
the EU authorized representative is:
Springer Nature Customer Service Center GmbH
Europaplatz 3, 69115 Heidelberg, Germany

Printed by Libri Plureos GmbH
in Hamburg, Germany